An
Introduction
to Clinical
Imaging

An Introduction to Clinical Imaging

D Lloyd Dixon
MB BS DDR FRCR FRACR MD
Honorary Consultant Radiologist, Alfred
Hospital, Melbourne; Associate in the Monash
Department of Surgery, Prince Henry's
Hospital, Melbourne

Leslie M Dugdale
MD ChB FRCR FRACR FRCP (Edin) FRACP
Chairman, Division of Diagnostic Imaging,
Queen Victoria Medical Centre, Melbourne

CHURCHILL LIVINGSTONE
MELBOURNE EDINBURGH LONDON AND
NEW YORK 1988

CHURCHILL LIVINGSTONE
Medical Division of Longman Group UK Limited

Distributed in the United States of America by Churchill
Livingstone Inc., 1560 Broadway, New York, N. Y. 10036,
and by associated companies, branches and representatives
throughout the world.

First published 1988

ISBN 0-443-03060-X

British Library Cataloguing in Publication Data
Dixon, D. Lloyd
  An introduction to clinical imaging
  1. Diagnostic imaging
  I. Title   II. Dugdale, Leslie M.
  616.07′54   RC78.7.D53
  ISBN 0-443-03662-4

Library of Congress Cataloging in Publication Data
Dixon, D. Lloyd.
  An introduction to clinical imaging.

  1. Diagnostic imaging.   I. Dugdale, Leslie M.
II. Title. [DNLM: 1. Nuclear Magnetic Resonance.
2. Radiography. 3. Radionuclide Imaging.
4. Tomography, X-Ray Computed. 5. Ultrasonic Diagnosis.
WN 200 D62li]
RC78.7.D53D59   1987   616.07′57   86-24487
ISBN 0-443-03662-4

Produced by Longman Singapore Publishers (Pte) Ltd.
Printed in Singapore

Preface

In recent years there has been a marked increase in imaging investigations available to clinicians with the introduction of ultrasound, computer tomography, nuclear medicine and magnetic resonance imaging. They have also seen the advent of interventional radiology.

The correct use of these entities is vital to the practice of good medicine. Many investigations overlap in the information they provide so that it is essential to know the indications, findings and limitations of the available organ imaging modalities to allow them to be best used, in association with clinical findings, to elucidate problems in medicine.

The many demands of the medical curriculum mean that there is usually insufficient time available for the student to gain an adequate knowledge of the use of these modalities.

The object of this book is to bridge this gap for the undergraduate and the recently graduated practitioner who in a given case will be required to choose the most appropriate investigation from the many available. To facilitate this, a selection of example problem-orientated flow charts giving the appropriate order in which investigations may best be performed have been included in addition to the findings of these investigations.

The method of presentation used in this text is the result of many years' experience in the teaching of students by the authors, and follows the lines that the students themselves have felt suited their needs best.

It is not claimed to be a complete textbook since the rare and many uncommon conditions are not dealt with, but only those which the user may expect to meet relatively commonly. As a basis for comparison the normal findings are described in addition to the pathological variations.

It is hoped that this book will fill a real need in the education of the undergraduate and will also be a useful reference later, after qualification, in the practice of clinical medicine.

Acknowledgements

The authors gratefully acknowledge the great help given by a number of people in the preparation of this book.

Professor Vernon C Marshall, Professor of Surgery, Monash University, provided great encouragement, generously supported us in a multitude of ways and also undertook the onerous task of proof-reading. Associate Professor J Freidin prepared all the line drawings except that of mediastinal masses which was taken from '*A Textbook of Radiology and Imaging*', permission to do so being generously granted by its editor, Dr David Sutton. The line drawings of fractures in the section on the skeletal system and those of pulmonary collapse in the respiratory section are based on drawings in the same text.

We also thank Dr John De Campo, Dr E Laufer, Dr J Martin, Dr John Pike, Dr Shirley Roberts, Dr Leon Slonim, Dr Sue Woodward and Dr Nina Zacharias for providing material for many illustrations and wish to acknowledge the late Dr H A Luke for his help in the same area.

M R I images were kindly provided by Professor W Hanafee of UCLA and Philips N V Eindhoven.

Mrs M Van Weel was tireless in typing the many drafts of the text. Ms Judy Waters of Churchill Livingstone was a guide and counsellor in many areas.

We owe a great debt to Kodak (A'asia) who generously provided the prints of all the illustrations, and especially to Dr W Fraser and Carol Hancock for their continuing interest and support. Mr Ross Genat exercised infinite care in the preparation of these prints.

Contents

1 Technology of Imaging

RADIOLOGY

X-RAYS

When electrons are accelerated across a vacuum tube by a high voltage and impinge on a tungsten target, part of their energy is converted to x-rays. When these rays are directed at a patient the different tissues attenuate them to varying degrees depending on the density and elemental composition of the tissue (see also 'Contrast media', page 3). The emergent x-rays are thus in a pattern called the 'radiation image'.

In a simple radiograph this radiation image is detected by a silver halide based film, the image being developed and fixed photographically (Figure 1.1). In other examinations the image is detected by a fluoroscopic screen (obsolete), image amplifier, xerographic plate, or digital detector.

Image amplifier

The emergent x-ray beam strikes a fluorescent screen from which the image is electronically amplified (Figure 1.2).

Xerography

The emergent beam strikes a plate coated with an electrically charged selenium layer. The x-rays discharge the various areas of the selenium to different degrees according to their attenuation. The varying charges on the plate are then developed by powder methods, the image being transferred to special paper for permanence. Soft tissues and in particular the breast are examined by this technique.

Digital detector

The radiation image is transformed to a numerical matrix which can be manipulated by a computer to increase or decrease brightness and contrast in the image, and to add or subtract

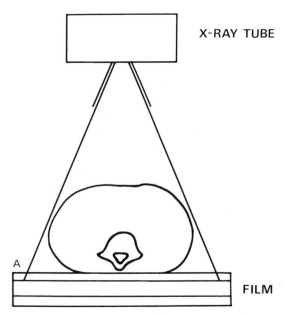

Fig. 1.1 (A) Principles of film radiography.
(B) Plain radiograph of abdomen.

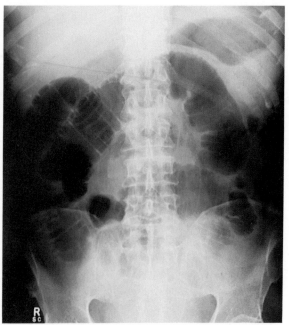

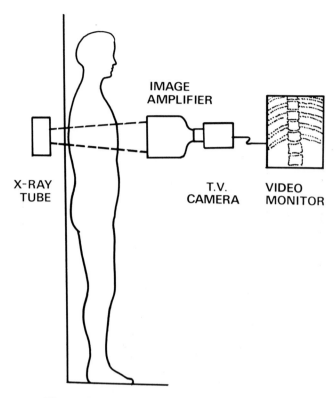

Fig. 1.2 Principles of fluoroscopy.

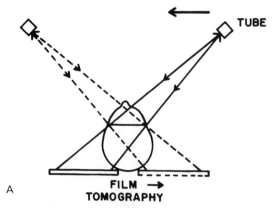

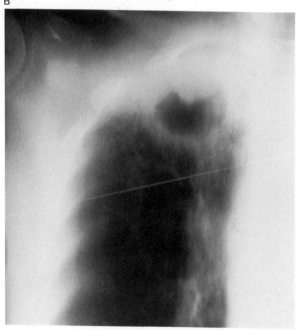

Fig. 1.3 (A) Principles of film tomography, with movement of x-ray tube and film.
(B) Tomograph of cavity at lung apex, with blurring out of overlying rib structures.

comparable images over time or by varying x-ray input. Digital subtraction angiography allows a considerably smaller dose of contrast medium to be used than in conventional angiography.

CONTRAST MEDIA

These are used to delineate the interior of many organs, blood vessels and lymphatics. The essential features of contrast media are that they have a different coefficient of absorption of x-rays relative to the surrounding tissues, being either more dense or less dense, and that they are non- toxic or of very low toxicity. Low density contrast media are gases used in double contrast studies of the gastrointestinal tract and in arthrography.

Examples of high density contrast media are barium sulphate, used in gastrointestinal examinations, and iodine compounds, used in examinations of the urinary tract and biliary systems. The iodine compounds are physiologically tailored to be excreted specifically by the liver or by the kidneys depending on the system that is to be opacified.

TOMOGRAPHY

By moving the x-ray tube and the film in opposite directions during an exposure (Figure 1.3) it is possible to show a thin slice of tissue delineated on the x-ray film. It has many uses, such as to display calcification, or cavitation within an area of lung opacity, or to show the contents of areas of sclerosis in bone.

COMPUTERIZED TOMOGRAPHY

Computerized tomography (CT) also depends on the differential absorption of radiation by various tissue types but the radiation image is detected by electronic methods and the signal converted to digital form. Radiation transmission measurements are obtained in multiple directions around the area of the patient in question and are converted by computer manipulation to an image (Figure 1.4). It is a highly sensitive examination and enables the display of very small differences in tissue density, e.g. that between the grey and white matter of the brain.

Computerized tomography has largely replaced techniques such as conventional tomography, air encephalography, and cerebral angiography. It reveals much information on the head and body not previously obtainable, and is a non-invasive technique.

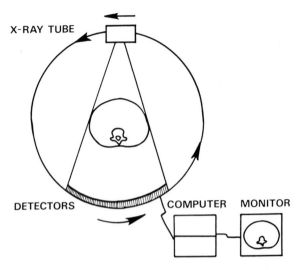

A

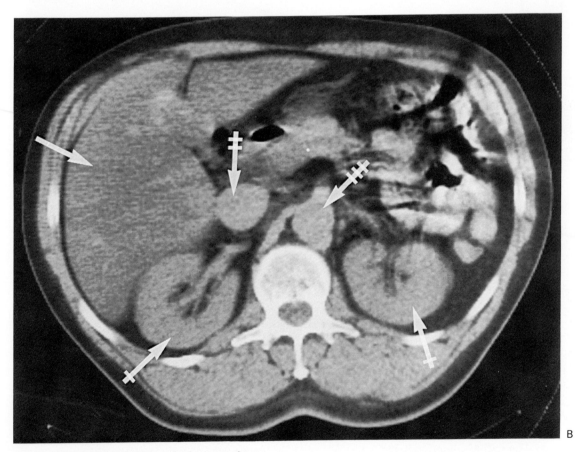

B

Fig. 1.4 (A) Principles of computerized tomography.
(B) CT scan of abdomen. Liver (→), kidneys (↔), inferior vena cava (⇥), aorta (⇥).

DIGITAL SUBTRACTION ANGIOGRAPHY

By subtracting a radiological background image from one in which the blood vessels have been opacified by contrast medium, the effective density of the contrast medium is enhanced. Computer acquisition and manipulation of digitalized image data enables refined, sensitive and safe angiography by either intravenous contrast injection or through very small intra-arterial catheters (Figure 1.5).

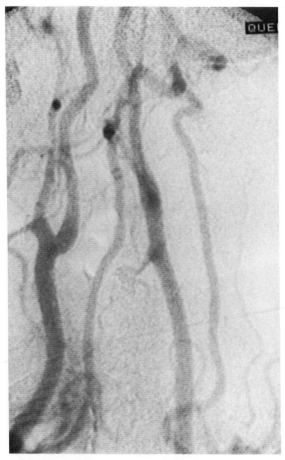

Fig. 1.5 Digital subtraction angiogram of the cervical arteries.

RADIOLOGICAL PROJECTIONS

For examinations of the skull, chest and extremities the minimal requirement is two films made at right angles to each other. The two views most commonly used are a postero-anterior view in which the x-ray beam passes from behind forwards through the structures examined, or an antero-posterior view in which the beam passes from front to back, and a lateral view in which the beam passes from one lateral aspect of the body through to the other lateral aspect (Figure 1.6). In addition to these basic views, many others, such as oblique views, may be required to show a region adequately.

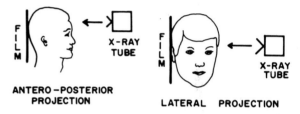

Fig. 1.6 Skull in two projections — AP and lateral.

FLUID LEVELS

These occur at the surface junction between a collection of liquid and overlying gas. They may be seen in abscess cavities, obstructed bowel and the accessory nasal sinuses. The fluid level, however, will be seen only when the x-ray beam passes parallel to the fluid surface (Figure 1.7). The patient must therefore be positioned so that this is possible, e.g. in the erect position to show fluid levels in the bowel.

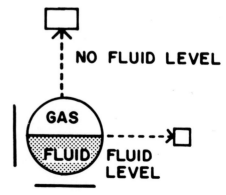

Fig. 1.7 Fluid levels can be seen only if the x-ray beam is horizontal and so parallel to the fluid interface surface.

ULTRASOUND

Although ultrasound is nominally sound of frequencies greater than audible, i.e. above 16 000 Hz, the frequencies used in medicine are usually in the 1–10 M Hz range. Short pulses of ultrasound from a transducer pass through the tissues with speeds and attenuation depending on the tissue density and elasticity. The attenuation is also dependent on the frequency of the sound. Reflection and scattering of the sound from tissue interfaces send a small proportion back to the transducer where it is converted to an electric voltage, varying proportionately to the detected sound intensity. This voltage is then amplified, stored, and displayed on a video screen in either graphical or image form (Figure 1.8).

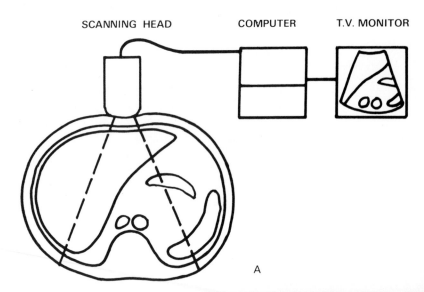

A

Fig. 1.8 (A) Principles of ultrasound imaging, using real-time sector system.
(B) Ultrasound scan of 28-week pregnancy.

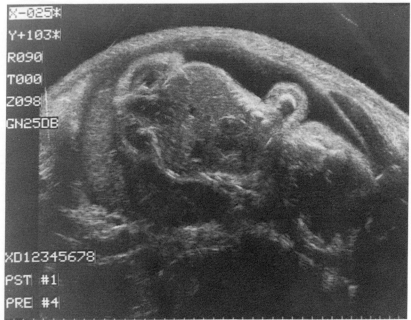

B

Ultrasound enables rapid accurate studies of anatomy, pathology and movement physiology of structures.

DOPPLER
The velocity of echo-producing objects moving toward or away from the transducer can be measured allowing the assessment of vascular stenoses or occlusions.

NUCLEAR MEDICINE

The common information source is the radiopharmaceutical which consists of two distinct parts:

1. The radionuclide, the source of high energy photons which carry the quantitative and positional information.

2. The pharmaceutical, which specifies the physiological and biochemical characteristics of the material.

The distribution and concentration of the radiopharmaceutical in space and time is detected and displayed or imaged usually by a gamma camera (Figure 1.9). Computer manipulation of spatial and temporal data provides dynamic assessment of physiological and biochemical processes.

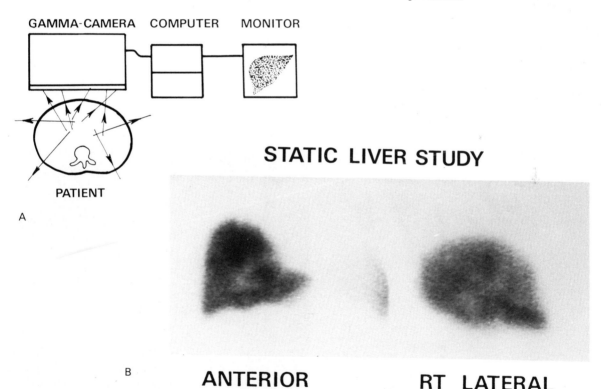

Fig. 1.9 (A) Principles of radionuclide scanning, using a gamma camera.
(B) Radionuclide liver scan, using technetium-99m labelled colloid.

THERMOGRAPHY

Skin temperature is assessed by a heat sensor which then displays the heat received as a temperature function either in colour or grey scale. Thermography has been used in the detection of breast lesions and vascular problems, but since skin temperature changes are not specific for any pathologies the technique is not widely used.

MAGNETIC RESONANCE IMAGING (MRI)

This relatively recently developed technique employs a strong magnetic field (about 1 000 times the earth's field) to align atomic nuclei with significant magnetic moments within an area of the patient's body (Figure 1.10a). These include hydrogen, sodium and phosphorus. The alignment is momentarily disturbed by a pulse of radio waves of the frequency (Larmor frequency) appropriate to the particular element under study, and the rate of return to the stable state is measured from the emission of radio waves. From this, images of elemental distribution can be produced (Figure 1.10b).

The absence of ionizing radiation renders the technique safe, and the very high quality of the anatomical and physiological data ensures that this will rapidly become a major imaging investigation.

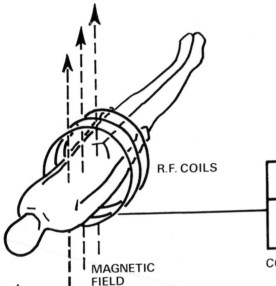

R.F. COILS

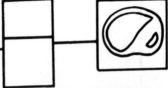

COMPUTER   MONITOR

MAGNETIC FIELD

A

Fig. 1.10 (A) Principles of magnetic resonance imaging. (B) MRI scan of pelvis, sagittal midline section, T1 weighted (Philips Gyroscan, by courtesy of Philips Medical Systems Div, Eindhoven, The Netherlands).

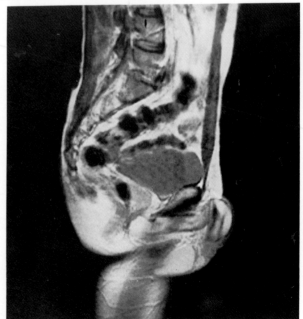

B

HAZARDS OF IMAGING

RADIATION RISKS
All x-ray or gamma radiation is ionizing and
hence potentially hazardous. The risks should in
all cases be balanced against the potential
benefits of the procedure. Rapidly growing
tissues are more sensitive to radiation than
others, so that lymphocytes with a half life of a
few days are much more sensitive than neurones
which are not replaced in adult life. Fetal tissue
is also very sensitive especially in the first
trimester of pregnancy. Radiation should be
avoided if possible during pregnancy. In general,
information should be sought on the date of the
last normal period, use of the contraceptive pill,
whether sterilization has been performed, the
patient's age, and other information factors
which will promote the sensible use of x-rays in
female patients.

Radiation of the gonads should be kept to a
minimum with the use, where possible, of lead
gonad shields and generally a reduction of
irradiated areas to a minimum in order to limit
scattered radiation. Computerized tomography
doses are generally small but should not be used
directly to gonads or fetal tissue.

Nuclear medicine procedures with internal
administration of radionuclides are generally of
low risk, although some techniques such as
brain scans and pancreas scans may give quite
high gonad doses. With modern equipment and
care, however, the risks of radiation damage are
exceedingly small.

ULTRASOUND
As yet no ill effects of ultrasound have been
discovered at diagnostic intensity levels — a
significant factor in the preference for ultrasound
in obstetrics when examining fetal tissue.

MAGNETIC RESONANCE IMAGING
The magnetic fields and electromagnetic pulses
have not been shown to cause any tissue
damage, and it is likely that the lack of ionizing
radiation will promote preferential utilization of
MRI in potentially hazardous situations.

PROCEDURAL HAZARDS
The aim of medical imaging is to produce
maximal information with minimal risk. The
advent of ultrasound, nuclear medicine, CT and
MRI is replacing many of the older invasive
investigations, such as pneumoencephalography
and many angiograms — and even the latter
may have their risk reduced by digital
subtraction angiography. Some hazards do,
however, remain but may be minimized by
proper application of the techniques by skilled
radiologists and by the correct choice and
sequence of examinations.

One of the prime purposes of this book is to
indicate the most appropriate examinations and
the order in which they should be requested and
performed in a given set of circumstances. If in
any doubt, proper consultation with the
radiologist, who is trained to assess potential
doses and risks and what are the most
appropriate examinations, is the best way to
reduce risks to the maximal advantage of the
patient.

2 Respiratory System

The chest

METHODS OF EXAMINATION

Plain radiographs

The minimal requirement for adequate radiological examination of the chest is two films, a *postero-anterior* (PA) projection (Figure 2.1a) and a *lateral* projection (Figure 2.1b). An adequately exposed postero-anterior view will show the dorsal vertebral bodies faintly through the heart shadow.

Tomography

This examination (see page 3) is valuable to demonstrate the presence of a cavity in the centre of an area of opacity, or to demonstrate the presence or absence of calcification within an opacity.

Bronchography

Contrast medium is introduced into the bronchi and the whole bronchial tree outlined (Figure 2.2). The greatest use of this examination is in demonstrating the presence of bronchiectasis but it is occasionally used to delineate broncho-stenotic lesions.

Radionuclide scanning

The distribution of the pulmonary artery blood flow may be indicated by the intravenous injection of labelled macro-aggregates (usually albumin) which embolize in the lung capillaries. The flow pattern is then shown by scanning.

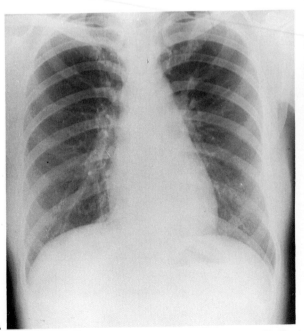

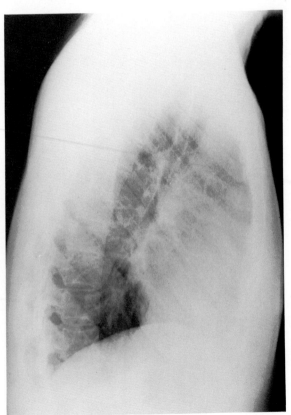

A   B

Fig. 2.1 (A) PA normal male chest. (B) Lateral normal male chest.

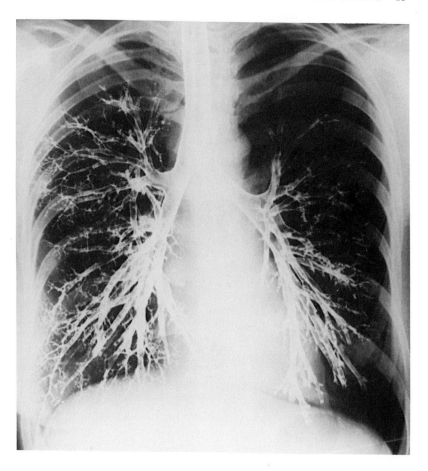

Fig. 2.2 Normal bronchogram.

Ventilation distribution may also be determined by scanning during the breathing of radioactive gas, usually ^{133}Xe. These techniques using a gamma camera to pick up and show the distribution of radiation are particularly useful in the detection of pulmonary embolism.

Computerized tomography
Cross-sectional tomography of the chest demonstrates well all the mediastinal, lung and chest wall structures. The absence of superimposed shadows permits high sensitivity, and the technique shows tumours, mediastinal nodes and pleural deposits particularly well.

Pulmonary angiography
Injection of radiographic contrast medium into the pulmonary artery via a cardiac catheter, or intravenously if subtraction angiography is used, permits radiography of the pulmonary vessels.

This technique is useful largely pre-operatively in cases of pulmonary embolism.

It is important to appreciate that medical imaging is an adjunct to history taking and clinical examination, and should not replace them. It is, however, sometimes misused, particularly in relation to chest examination. In cases, for example, of cardiac failure or pneumonia, after an initial chest radiograph the course of the condition should be followed by clinical examination and not by multiple radiographs if the patient is improving. Only when there is clinical doubt about the patient's progress are further radiographs warranted, except for a final check film. The replacement of clinical examination by radiographs under these and similar conditions gives unnecessary irradiation of the patient, adds significantly to the rising costs of medical services, and adds little to the assessment of the patient's condition.

THE NORMAL CHEST

Displacement or alteration in the shape or size of normal structures can be an important indication of the type of pathology present. An understanding of the normal appearances is therefore important, and a routine of examination should be developed so that all visible structures are examined even when there is an obvious lesion present.

THE POSTERO-ANTERIOR VIEW (Figure 2.3)

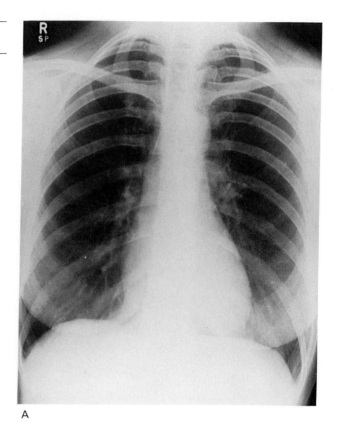

Fig. 2.3 (A) PA normal female chest.
         (B) Diagram of principal landmarks of PA chest.

A

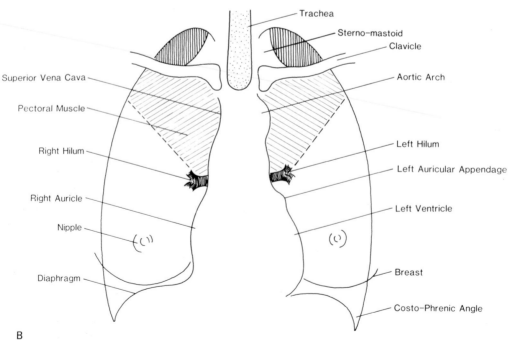

B

Chest wall

Muscle shadows

At the apex of each lung above the clavicle the sterno-mastoid casts an opaque shadow adjacent to the spine with a well-defined concave lateral margin. The pectoral muscles overlie the upper half of the chest below the clavicle, and cause slight loss of translucency of the chest over the area. This loss of translucency has a well defined lower edge which runs upwards and outwards towards the head of the humerus.

Breast and nipple shadows

The female breasts produce areas of diminished translucency (which increase in degree from above downwards) over the lower half of the lung fields. Depending on the size of the breasts there will be a sharply defined convex lower margin to the shadow either above or below the level of the diaphragm.

The nipples may produce a small round soft opacity over the lower part of each lung field and can be recognized because the opacity is usually bilateral and symmetrically placed.

Bone shadows

The shadows of the clavicles and ribs are easily recognized. The costal cartilages are normally not visible on a radiograph but are visible as mottled opacities when calcified.

Lung landmarks

Trachea

The trachea can be identified in the PA view as a narrow band of translucency approximately 1.5–2 cm in width overlying the lower cervical and upper dorsal vertebrae. It lies in the midline and as a result the spinous processes of the vertebrae can be seen through its shadow. Any deviation of the trachea from the midline is abnormal.

Diaphragm

The two domes of the diaphragm are convex upwards with the right dome being usually 1–3 cm higher than the left dome. At its highest point the right dome reaches the tenth rib in the mid-clavicular line on full inspiration in the average person; but the patient's habitus does affect the height of the diaphragm, which lies at a higher level in the sthenic and at a lower level in the asthenic person. Occasionally the diaphragm will have humps on its contour but these are usually normal findings.

Costo-phrenic angles

In the PA projection the diaphragm meets the lateral chest wall at an acute angle on each side. These are called the lateral costo-phrenic angles. Obliteration of these angles is abnormal.

Mediastinum

The shadow cast by the mediastinum is made up for the most part by the heart. The heart shadow projects more to the left than to the right of the midline — approximately one-third of the shadow lies to the right of the midline. The margins of the mediastinal shadow are sharply defined. The left margin, when traced from above downwards, shows a bulge (due to the aortic arch) a short distance below the inner ends of the clavicles. A short distance below this is a second but less pronounced bulge due to the main pulmonary artery, with sometimes a third small bulge below this due to the appendage of the left atrium. Below this point the smooth convexity of the heart shadow is formed by the left ventricle.

The right mediastinal margin is formed from above downwards by the slightly concave shadow of the superior vena cava and below this by the smooth convexity of the right atrium. The heart size is within normal limits if the greatest transverse diameter of the heart shadow is equal to, or less than, half the greatest transverse diameter of the thorax.

Hilar shadows

The shadows of the hila of the lungs are made up for the most part by the right and left branches of the pulmonary artery which can be seen to branch as the vessels run out into the lung fields. Lymph nodes and pulmonary veins make up the relatively small remaining amount of the hilar shadows. The left hilar shadow normally lies approximately 1 cm higher than the right. The two hilar shadows are of equal size.

Fissures
The pleura is invisible on ordinary radiographs except where it is reflected over the mediastinum and where it dips into the fissures between the lobes of the lung, where it can sometimes be seen as a fine white line. On the right side the transverse fissure between the upper and middle lobes runs horizontally from the junction of the upper third and lower two-thirds of the hilar shadow to the lateral chest wall (Figure 2.4).

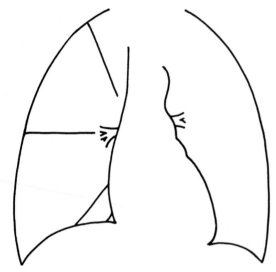

Fig. 2.4 Diagram of position of normal pleural fissures in PA projection.

This is an important landmark when visible, but may normally run slightly upwards or slightly downwards as it is traced laterally. The oblique fissures are invisible on the PA radiograph. Occasionally an oblique fine white line is seen running downwards and inwards to the mediastinal shadow from the region of the lung apex on the right side; this represents a fissure caused by the azygos vein which has pulled down through the lung to the region just above the hilum. A further fissure may sometimes be seen at the right base as a fine white line running upwards and inwards to the heart shadow from the diaphragm; this represents a

fissure which separates a small segment of lung from the remainder of the lung.

Lung markings
The bronchi are not visible on the radiograph unless they are seen end on, when they show as small ring shadows. These ring shadows are generally adjacent to a small round opacity which represents the accompanying blood vessel seen end on. The pulmonary markings are therefore due to the shadows of the branches of pulmonary arteries and veins. These branch and taper as they run peripherally from the hilum and extend right out the lateral chest wall. It is not possible to distinguish arteries from veins except possibly in the right lower lung field where some veins run horizontally to the heart.

THE LATERAL VIEW (Figure 2.5)
There is little difference in the appearances of the chest in the two lateral views.

Chest wall

Spine
The first vertebral body seen clearly at the upper end of the spinal shadow is usually that of the second dorsal vertebra.

Ribs
The ribs on the two sides overlap each other in the lateral view making identification of individual ribs difficult.

Sternum
In adults the sternum usually appears as a single, slightly convex shadow anteriorly; but the manubrio-sternal joint may be visible. In children the sternum is seen to be made up of a series of ossification centres with gaps between them due to uncalcified cartilage.

Lung landmarks

Trachea
The trachea can be seen as a band of translucency 1.5–2 cm in diameter running

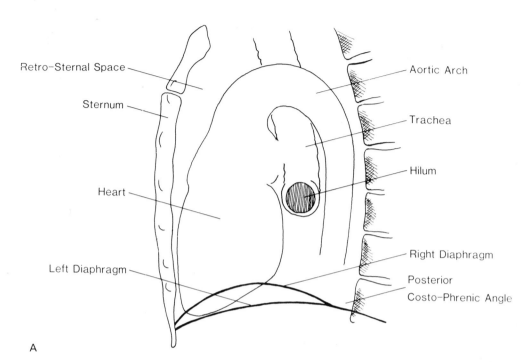

Retro-Sternal Space
Sternum
Heart
Left Diaphragm

Aortic Arch
Trachea
Hilum
Right Diaphragm
Posterior
Costo-Phrenic Angle

A

Fig. 2.5 (A) Diagram of principal landmarks of lateral chest.
(B) Lateral normal female chest.

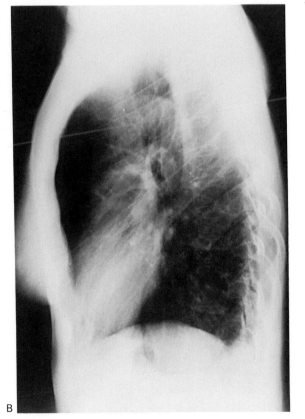

B

vertically downwards or inclined slightly
backwards, a short distance in front of the
dorsal spine. The shadow ends at the hilum,
where a large ring shadow may be seen
representing a main bronchus seen end on.

Diaphragm
The two domes of the diaphragm should be
visible and the left dome may be recognized if
there is gas in the fundus of the stomach
beneath it. Due to projection, the dome closest
to the film usually appears to be higher and
smaller than the other dome. A hump on the
anterior part of the right dome is often seen and
is a normal finding.

Costo-phrenic angles
Each dome of the diaphragm meets the posterior
chest wall at an acute angle to form the
posterior costo-phrenic angle which is normally
clear and air-containing.

Mediastinum

The two hilar shadows overlie each other and are not recognizable as separate entities. The bulk of the mediastinal shadow is made up of the shadow of the heart in the lower half of the chest. The shadow of the anterior wall of the heart is often fused with the sternum in its lower part, but in its upper part it swings convexly away from the sternum and the aortic arch can usually be identified arising from the heart and curving backwards. The posterior margin of the heart shadow is convex and sharply defined. The shadows of the heart and diaphragm fuse where they meet.

Fissures

In the left lateral view the oblique fissure between the left upper and lower lobes may be seen as a thin white line commencing above at the level of the fourth dorsal vertebra and running downwards and forwards through the hilar shadow to end below 2–5 cm behind the junction of diaphragm and sternum (Figure 2.6). In the right lateral view the oblique fissure between the right upper and middle lobes and the lower lobe runs from the region of the fourth dorsal vertebra through the hilum and terminates where the diaphragm meets the sternum (Figure 2.7). In this view the horizontal fissure may also be seen as a thin white line running forwards from the hilum to the sternum. Slight variations in the position of these fissures are within normal limits but significant shift in their position is a most important diagnostic sign.

Lung markings

In the lateral view the markings in the two lungs overlie each other with the result that individual markings are very difficult to identify.

Retrosternal window

Behind the upper half of the sternum there is a clear area called the retrosternal window, which is bounded posteriorly by the aorta and upper half of the heart shadow. It is bounded below by the junction of the heart shadow with the sternum.

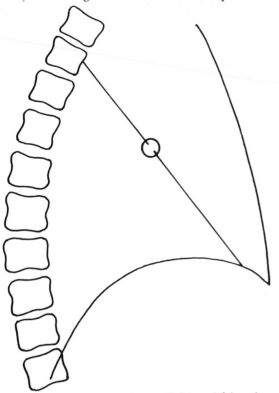

Fig. 2.6 Diagram of pleural fissure of left lung, left lateral view.

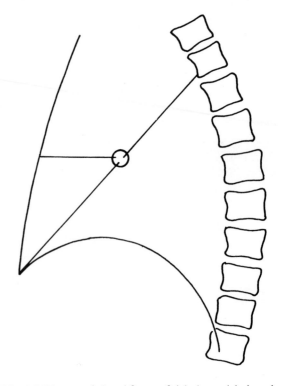

Fig. 2.7 Diagram of pleural fissure of right lung, right lateral view.

LESIONS OF THE PLEURA

The pleura is not normally visible on the radiograph except sometimes in those situations, such as the lung fissures and mediastinal reflection of the pleura, where the pleura is seen end on and appears as a thin white line on the radiograph.

PLEURAL FLUID

The presence of fluid in the pleural cavity can be recognized, but it is not possible from the radiographic appearances to distinguish the type of fluid present. Transudate, exudate, blood and pus all produce the same appearance.

Pleural fluid always collects in the most dependent part of the pleural cavity unless prevented from doing so by pleural adhesions. Although very small collections of pleural fluid of the order of 10–15 cm^3 can be recognized using special techniques it would seem that it requires 200–300 cm^3 to be present before it is recognizable on the standard PA and lateral views.

With the patient in the erect position a small effusion of 200–300 cm^3 will therefore be recognized by the obliteration of the posterior costo-phrenic angle. As the amount of fluid increases the lateral costo-phrenic angle will become obliterated (Figure 2.8). With larger amounts of fluid, an area of opacity appears over the lower part of the lung field. This area of opacity will be seen to extend to its highest level adjacent to the lateral chest wall in the PA view

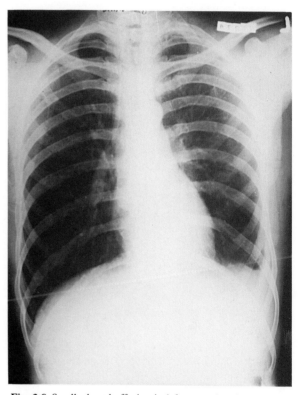

Fig. 2.8 Small pleural effusion in left costo-phrenic angle.

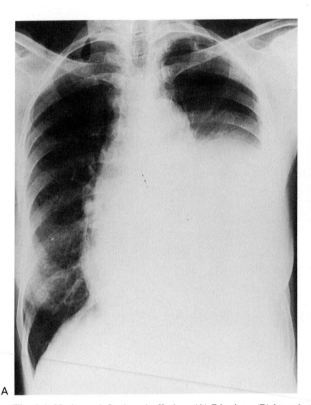 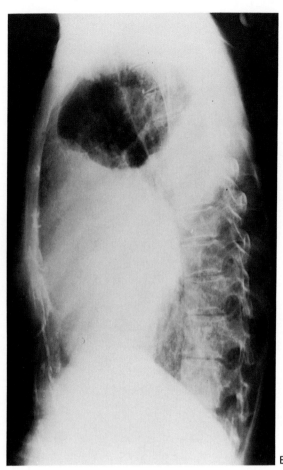

Fig. 2.9 Moderate left pleural effusion: (A) PA view; (B) lateral view.

(Figure 2.9) and the anterior and posterior chest walls in the lateral view. In the lateral view the fluid, as well as extending up the anterior and posterior chest walls, may enter and extend up into the oblique fissure.

In fact the fluid surrounds the anterior, lateral and posterior surfaces of the lung evenly at the same height but since the x-ray beam passes through a thicker collection in the lateral part of the chest than it does elsewhere the fluid here casts a denser shadow and appears to extend up the lateral chest wall (Figure 2.10).

When the fluid appears to extend up along the chest wall the shadow has a slightly concave margin on the aspect next to the lung. With a massive collection of fluid in the pleural cavity there is complete opacity of the hemithorax with associated displacement of the trachea and mediastinum towards the opposite side (Figure 2.11).

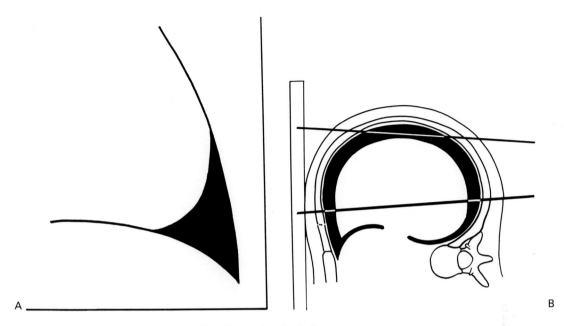

Fig. 2.10 (A) Diagram of appearance of moderate pleural effusion.
(B) Diagram of cross-section of chest with pleural effusion, showing apparent extra density at lateral wall of chest.

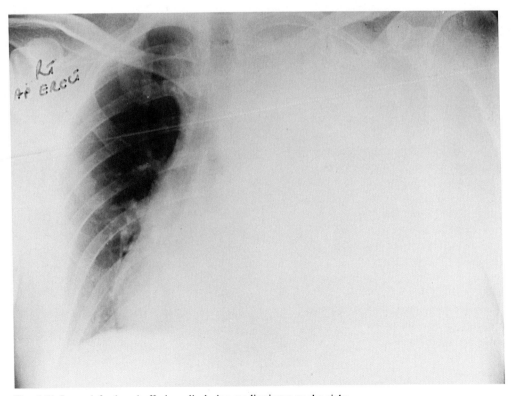

Fig. 2.11 Large left pleural effusion, displacing mediastinum to the right.

Sometimes fluid will become encysted in a fissure. In the oblique fissures such an encysted effusion appears as an ill-defined area of opacity in the PA view, but in the lateral view will be seen to be sharply defined and biconvex in shape.

An encysted effusion in the transverse fissure is seen as a sharply defined, biconvex opacity in both the PA and lateral views (Figure 2.12).

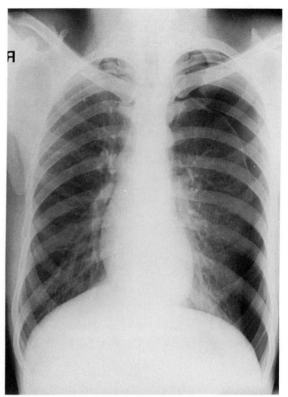

Fig. 2.13 Moderate left-sided pneumothorax.

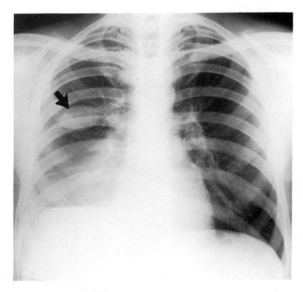

Fig. 2.12 Encysted effusion in right horizontal fissure ($\rightarrow$).

PNEUMOTHORAX
In the normal chest the pulmonary markings extend from the hilum to the chest wall.

When air is present in the pleural cavity there is an absence of lung markings, in the PA view, in the area occupied by the air. This area is also more radiolucent than the area occupied by the lung. The margins of the partially contracted lung may also be seen (Figure 2.13).

TENSION PNEUMOTHORAX
If a ball-valve mechanism is operating at the site where air is entering the pleural cavity a tension pneumothorax may develop.

Radiological appearances (Figure 2.14)
1. Marked hypertranslucency of the hemithorax.

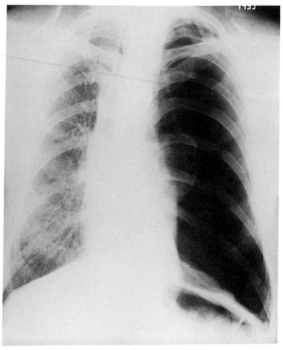

Fig. 2.14 Tension pneumothorax displacing mediastinum.

2. The collapsed lung lying as an opacity at the hilum.

3. Displacement of the trachea and mediastinum towards the opposite side.

4. Downward displacement and flattening of the diaphragm on the affected side.

5. Widened intercostal spaces with the ribs running more horizontally on the affected side.

PLEURAL CALCIFICATION

Dense linear plaques of calcification may be seen on the pleural surfaces (Figure 2.15). These may result from a number of pathological conditions, the most common of which are old empyema, old haemothorax, asbestosis and silicosis.

PLEURAL NEOPLASMS

All pleural tumours tend to present as well-defined opacities with a broad base to the chest wall. Induction of a pneumothorax may be necessary to decide whether the tumour lies in the lung or the pleura.

Metastases
The most common pleural tumour and may be single or multiple.

Primary tumours
Benign tumours such as fibromas do occur but are rare.

Mesothelioma is the most common *malignant* tumour and is often associated with asbestosis. It is a reasonably common tumour. The tumour

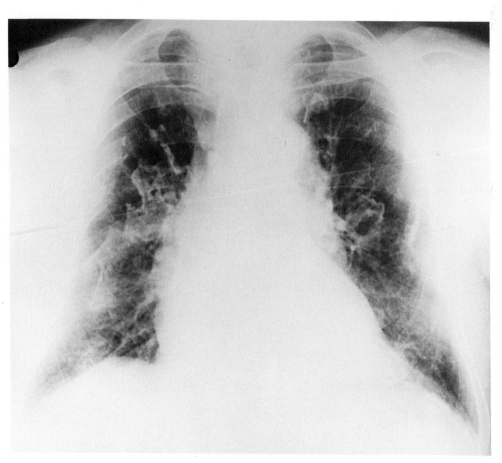

Fig. 2.15 Pleural calcification in asbestosis.

shows as an opacity with a smooth surface and is adjacent to the chest wall (Figure 2.16).

Computerized tomography shows pleural lesions particularly well (Figure 2.17).

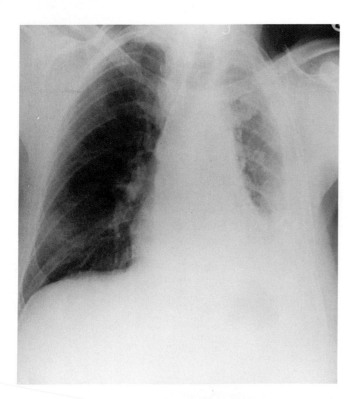

Fig. 2.16 Pleural thickening, on left.

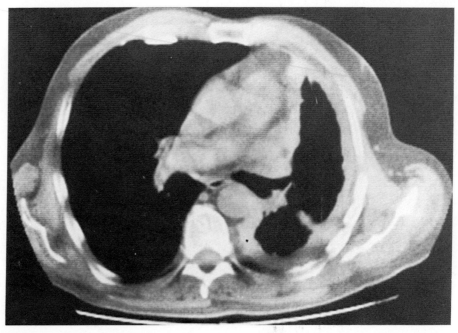

Fig. 2.17 CT of chest showing gross pleural thickening.

LESIONS OF THE LUNGS

WHOLE LUNG COLLAPSE

Radiological appearances (Figure 2.18)
  1. Complete opacity of the hemithorax.
  2. Displacement of the trachea and
mediastinal contents towards the side of the
collapse.
  3. Narrowing of the intercostal spaces and
greater obliquity of ribs on the side of the
collapsed lung.

LOBAR COLLAPSE

Radiological appearances common to all lobes
  1. Reduced volume of the lobe.
  2. Opacity of the lobe.
  3. Displacement of fissures towards the
opaque lobe.
  4. Vascular shadows in the remainder of the
lung are more widely spread than normal.

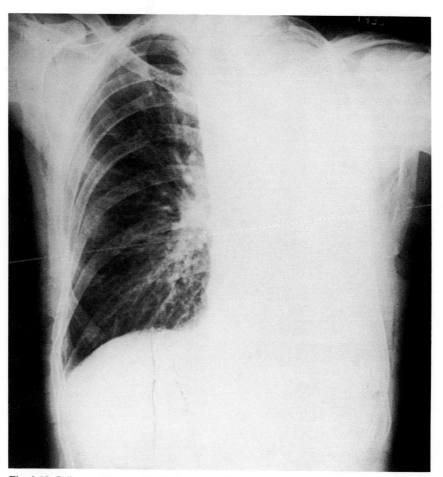

Fig. 2.18 Collapse of lung, with displacement of mediastinum towards the affected side.

Right upper lobe collapse (Figure 2.19)

The PA view

1. The transverse fissure, if visible, runs obliquely upwards towards the apex of the lung.
2. There is an area of opacity in the upper part of the hemithorax adjacent to the mediastinum.
3. The trachea deviates slightly to the right.
4. The right hilar shadow is slightly elevated.

The right lateral view

There is an area of opacity with sharply defined margins lying in the midpart of the upper half of the chest.

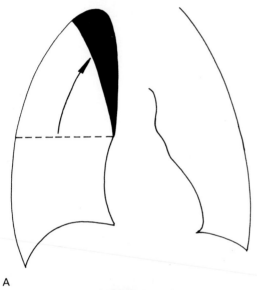

A

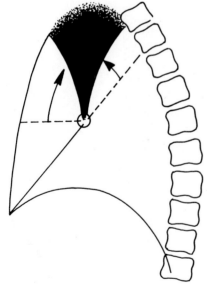

B

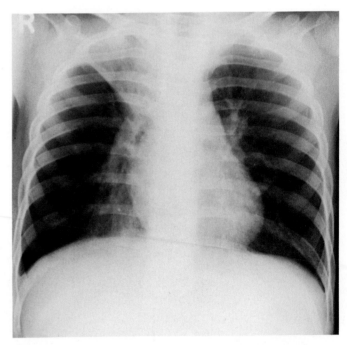

C

Fig. 2.19 Diagrams of pattern of collapse of right upper lobe:
(A) PA projection;
(B) lateral projection showing shift of fissures.
(C) PA radiograph of right upper lobe collapse.

Right middle lobe collapse

The PA view

1. There may only be a vague loss of translucency adjacent to the lower part of the heart shadow.

2. If the transverse fissure is visible it runs downwards and outwards from the hilum (Figure 2.20a, c).

The right lateral view

There is a triangular area of opacity with sharply defined margins running downwards and forwards from the hilum (Figure 2.20b, d).

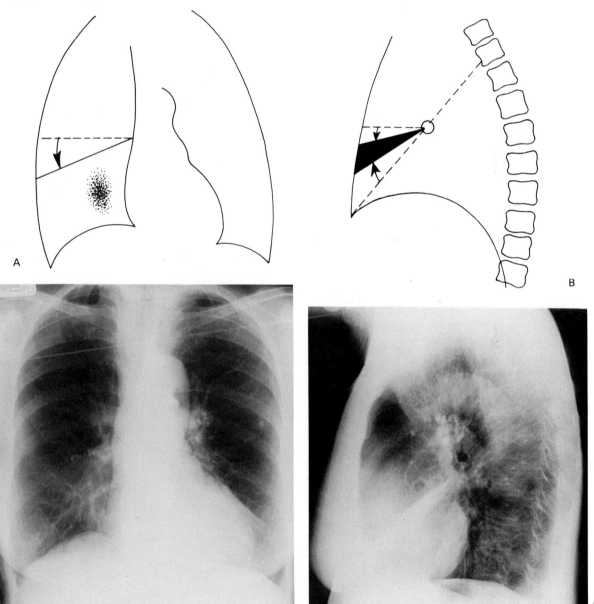

Fig. 2.20 Diagrams of pattern of right middle lobe collapse: (A) PA projection; (B) lateral projection. Radiographs of chest with right middle lobe collapse: (C) PA projection; (D) lateral projection.

Right lower lobe collapse

The PA view
1. There is an area of opacity at the base of the lung adjacent to the heart shadow with a well-defined lateral margin.
2. The transverse fissure, if visible, runs downwards and outwards from the hilum (Figure 2.21a).

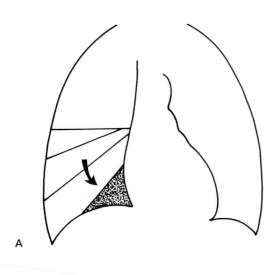

A

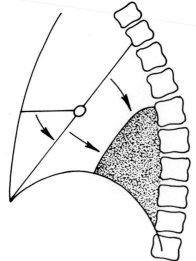

B

Fig. 2.21 Diagrams of pattern of right lower lobe collapse:
(A) PA projection;
(B) lateral projection.

The right lateral view
1. There is an area of opacity overlying the posterior portion of the lower half of the chest. This opacity has a sharply defined anterior margin because it is bounded anteriorly by the oblique fissure which has become displaced posteriorly (Figure 2.21b).
2. The transverse fissure if visible now runs downwards and forwards from the hilum.

Left upper lobe collapse

The PA view
There is an area of opacity in the left lung field adjacent to the mediastinum in the upper half of the chest and this area has an ill-defined margin (Figure 2.22a).

The lateral view
There is a band of opacity with a sharply defined posterior margin lying behind the sternum (Figure 2.22b). The sharply defined posterior margin is due to the oblique fissure which has moved forward as the lobe has collapsed.

Left lower lobe collapse

The PA view
There is a triangular area of opacity which can be seen through the heart shadow to the left of the midline and adjacent to the spine (Figure 2.23a).

The lateral view
There is an area of opacity at the base posteriorly which has a sharply defined anterior margin due to the left oblique fissure which has become displaced backwards (Figure 2.23b).

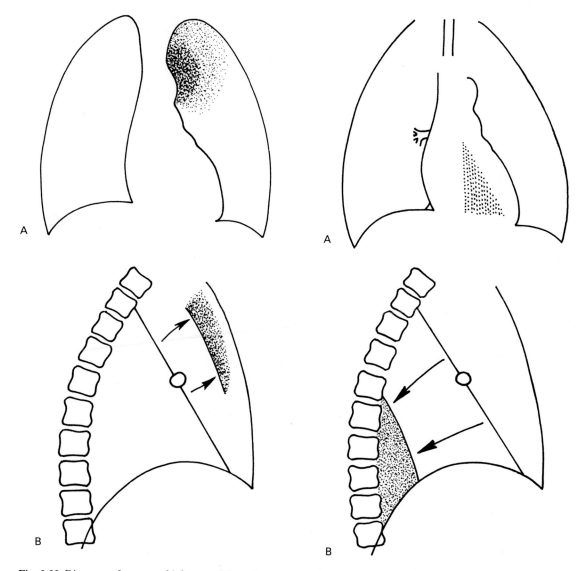

Fig. 2.22 Diagrams of pattern of left upper lobe collapse:
(A) PA projection;
(B) lateral projection.

Fig. 2.23 Diagrams of pattern of left lower lobe collapse:
(A) PA projection;
(B) lateral projection.

PLATE-LIKE ATELECTASIS

Radiological appearances
Plate-like areas of atelectasis appear as linear areas of opacity several centimetres long and 2–3 mm in diameter (Figure 2.24). They usually occur in the basal regions of the lungs and are roughly horizontal. They are seen in cases with limited diaphragmatic movement and are frequently seen after abdominal operations. They are most probably due to obstruction of small bronchi by secretion and tend to be of a transient nature.

SEGMENTAL ATELECTASIS

Radiological appearances
Segmental atelectasis appears as a wedge-shaped area of opacity with its apex towards the hilum and its base on the pleura. It results from obstruction of a bronchus by carcinoma, foreign body, or similar obstructive lesions.

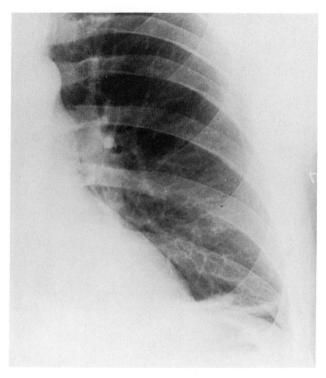

Fig. 2.24 Plate-like atelectasis at left base.

PULMONARY CONSOLIDATION

Consolidation of the lungs takes two forms. It may be lobar, and uniformly involve the whole or portion of a lobe; or it may be scattered throughout the affected part of the lung in small areas of bronchopneumonia.

The hilar nodes are not usually enlarged in cases of simple pneumonia. Areas of pneumonia do not tend to increase in extent after they have been demonstrated and, although some simple pneumonias are slow to clear, delay in resolution or enlarged hilar nodes should make one very suspicious that there is a pre-existing lesion present such as bronchiectasis or carcinoma of a bronchus. Some pneumonias, notably staphylococcal pneumonia, tend to break down and produce cavities; in the case of staphylococcal pneumonia these cavities are thin walled and may persist after resolution of the consolidation (Figure 2.25).

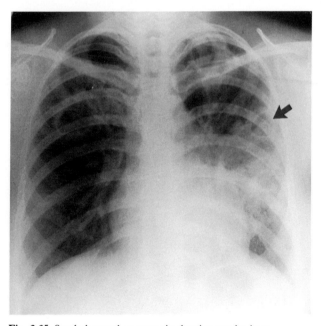

Fig. 2.25 Staphylococcal pneumonia showing patchy lung consolidation, with early cavity formation (→).

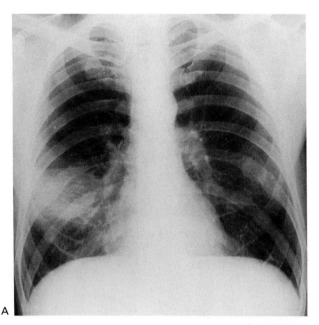

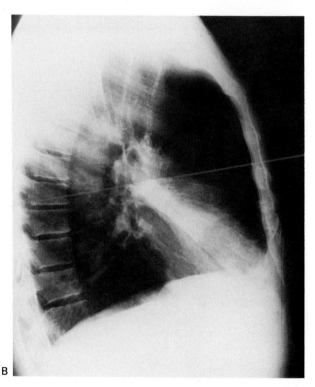

Lobar pneumonia

Radiological appearances

1. An area of uniform opacity confined within the boundaries of the lobe.

2. There is often associated slight loss of volume of the affected lobe (Figure 2.26).

3. No evidence of vascular markings can be seen within the area.

4. Frequently air-filled bronchi can be seen as translucent areas within the opacity: the so-called 'air bronchogram'.

5. If the whole lobe is involved the margins of the opacity are well-defined because the fissures confine the process.

6. If only part of a lobe is involved then the same appearances are seen but the margins of the opacity are ill-defined unless the process lies against one of the fissures.

In acute pulmonary inflammation there may be only a generalized increase in pulmonary markings in the area involved, and no uniform consolidation.

Pneumonic changes in the lung may be accompanied by fluid in the pleural cavity.

Fig. 2.26 Lobar pneumonia involving right middle lobe:
(A) PA projection;
(B) lateral projection.

Bronchopneumonia

This condition may arise *de novo* but is also seen postoperatively or following aspiration of material.

Radiological appearances

1. Increased markings in the area involved.
2. Small, ill defined areas of opacity due to localized areas of consolidation (Figure 2.27).

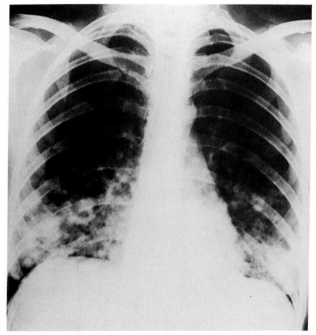

Fig. 2.27 Bilateral basal bronchopneumonia, with patchy consolidation.

LUNG ABSCESS

Lung abscesses usually develop in a pre-existing area of consolidation and, most commonly, in an area of consolidation distal to bronchial obstruction from such causes as carcinoma, inhaled foreign body, or an adenoma. Some types of pneumonia, particularly those due to the *Staphylococcus* or *Friedlander's bacillus*, are more prone to break down and form abscesses than are other types.

Radiological appearances

When an abscess occurs in an area of consolidation beyond a bronchial obstruction there is usually an element of collapsed lung present in association with the lesion. In such cases enlargement of hilar nodes should be looked for because a common cause for such appearances is a carcinoma of the bronchus. *There are no enlarged nodes with a simple lung abscess.* The presence of an abscess is recognized by the appearance of a gas containing area within the area of consolidation (Figure 2.28).

BRONCHIECTASIS

This condition may rarely be congenital but more commonly follows whooping cough or

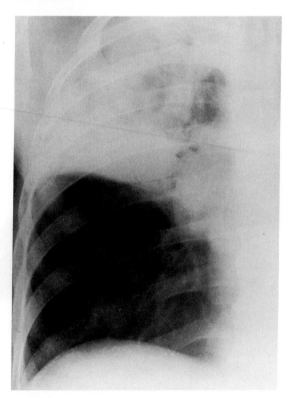

Fig. 2.28 Consolidation in right upper zone, breaking down to form a lung abscess.

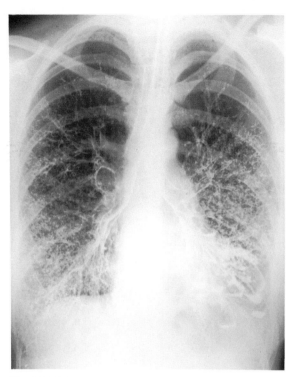

Fig. 2.29 Bilateral basal bronchiectasis, shown by bronchography.

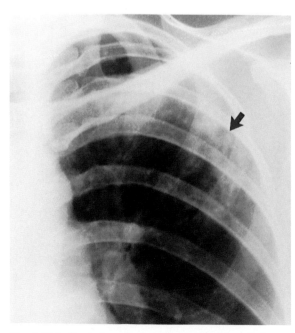

Fig. 2.30 Left apical opacity (→) due to early tuberculosis.

measles in childhood when segments of pulmonary atelectasis occur, followed by fibrosis and subsequent dilatation of the bronchi. It is frequently associated with chronic sinusitis.

Radiological appearances
1. Plain radiographs:
(a) there may be no abnormality;
(b) there may be increased markings in the basal areas;
(c) there may be recurrent episodes of consolidation, usually at the base of a lung.
2. Bronchography: the dilated bronchi are demonstrated and this is the only certain method of making the diagnosis (Figure 2.29).

PRIMARY PULMONARY TUBERCULOSIS
This occurs in children and adults who have had no previous infection with tuberculosis.

Radiological appearances
1. Consolidation: usually a small area, but which may be extensive and which can occur anywhere in the lung fields.
2. Node enlargement: the hilar nodes on the side of the lesion are enlarged and this enlargement, which is sometimes very marked, may extend to involve most of the mediastinal nodes. With healing the nodes return to normal size but occasionally calcify.
3. Ghon's focus: with healing, resolution of the area of consolidation is usually complete, but a small calcified nodule, the Ghon's focus, may persist after healing.

SECONDARY TUBERCULOSIS
This occurs in people who have at some time had a primary tuberculous infection.

Radiological appearances
Secondary tuberculous *consolidation* almost invariably occurs in the posterior part of the lung apex. It may appear initially as a collection of small, discrete areas, or as an ill-defined, soft, rounded area of opacity (Figure 2.30). It may be bilateral or unilateral. There is *no* associated node enlargement. These appearances are almost diagnostic of a tuberculous infection.

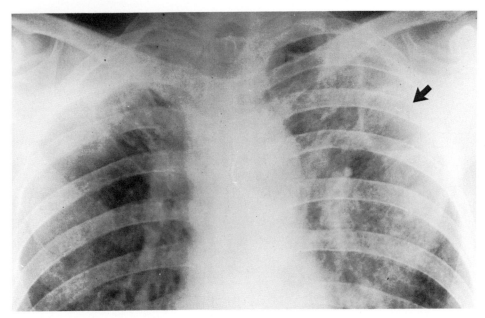

Fig. 2.31 Bilateral chronic apical tuberculosis, with cavity in left upper zone (→).

Subsequent changes

1. Healing: the area of consolidation may resolve and leave only a small fibrous scar.

2. Cavitation: central necrosis may occur and lead to the formation of a cavity which appears as an area of translucency, sometimes with a fluid level, within the area of consolidation. If the surrounding consolidation clears, the cavity will be seen to have a relatively thin wall and an irregular inner surface (Figure 2.31). There is usually evidence of fibrosis in the surrounding lung.

3. Fibrosis: an irregular increase in lung markings may appear in the apical area associated with elevation of the hilum on that side (Figure 2.32), and on the right side elevation of the transverse fissure. These changes are the result of fibrous tissue forming in the area of chronic infection and as the fibrous tissue contracts it pulls on the hilum and fissure, which are movable. Marked fibrosis may result in an increase in translucency of the remainder of the lung due to overdistension to compensate for the loss of volume of the upper part of the lung.

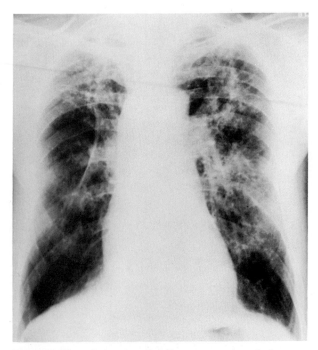

Fig. 2.32 Bilateral chronic apical fibrocaseous tuberculosis, showing reduction of upper lobe volume, and elevation of lung hila.

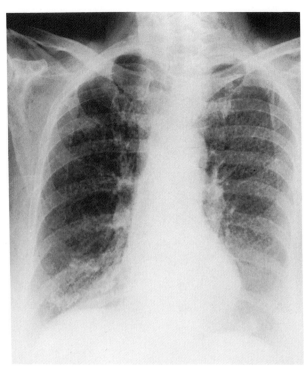

Fig. 2.33 Miliary tuberculosis.

4. Calcification: tuberculous foci frequently undergo central caseation and this caseous material may become calcified. This usually results in aggregations of calcification, with uncalcified foci visible in the surrounding lung. In chronic tuberculous disease there may be any combination of consolidation, fibrosis, cavitation, and calcification.

5. Miliary nodulation: involvement of a blood vessel by a tuberculous focus may lead to haematogenous spread of bacilli. In the lungs there is a uniform involvement of both lungs by tiny (1–2 mm) soft nodules thickly scattered so that the lung areas on the radiograph assume a grey appearance (Figure 2.33).

6. Tuberculoma: a small rounded opacity (1–3 cm) with a rather well-defined edge, which may occur anywhere in the lung and frequently contains specks of calcification (Figure 2.34). There are often small satellite foci in the area and there may be linear markings running towards the hilum from the region of the opacity.

Appearances similar to both primary and secondary pulmonary tuberculosis may be caused by coccidiomycosis and histoplasmosis, fungus diseases which are endemic in parts of America.

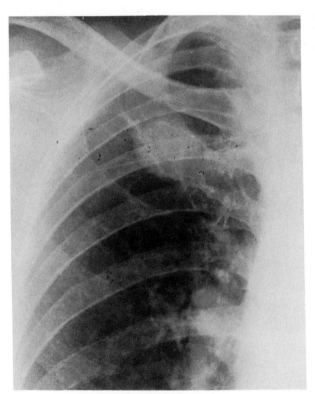

Fig. 2.34 Tuberculoma presenting as a right apical coin lesion.

MYCETOMA

Inhalation of *Aspergillus* fungus may lead to the following:

1. Transient but recurrent areas of consolidation in the lungs.

2. Mycelia collecting as a mass in a pre-existing cavity in the lung (mycetoma) (Figure 2.35). The mass is mobile and will alter its position in the cavity with alterations in the posture of the patient, which helps to differentiate it from two other conditions which can give a similar appearance of a mass in a cavity: (a) blood clot in a cavity, (b) cavitating neoplasm.

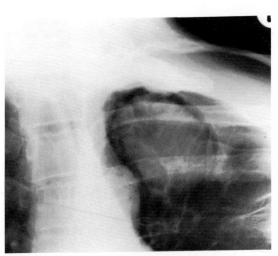

Fig. 2.35 Mycetoma presenting as a mycelial ball in a thin-walled lung cavity.

PULMONARY TRAUMA

Pulmonary contusion

This is the result of blunt trauma to the chest and can occur in the absence of rib fractures.

Radiological appearances

1. Irregular, ill-defined, scattered areas of consolidation, or a larger homogeneous area of consolidation which may be bilateral even though the trauma affected only one side (Figure 2.36). These areas appear within a few hours of the trauma.

2. Resolution occurs within a few days.

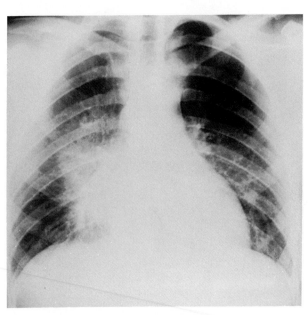

Fig. 2.36 Right pulmonary opacity due to contusion. There are also minor changes at the left base.

Pulmonary haematoma and traumatic lung cyst

These may also follow blunt trauma within a few hours, particularly if the lung has been torn.

Radiological appearances

1. Very thin-walled air cysts (pneumatoceles) which may or may not contain an air-fluid level.

2. A rounded area of opacity which is the result of haemorrhage (pulmonary haematoma) (Figure 2.37).

These changes tend to persist for long periods and may still be visible several months after injury.

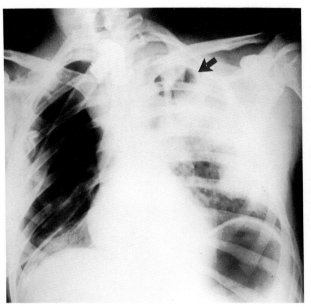

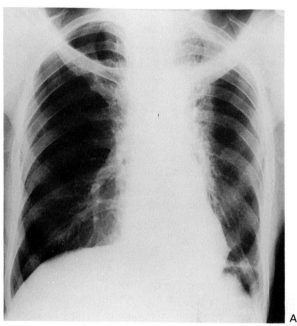

Fig. 2.37 Left apical post-traumatic lung cyst in massively contused left lung (→).

Radiation injury
The onset of radiological changes in acute irradiation pneumonitis occurs at the earliest one to two months after the course of radiation is completed and may be delayed for several months.

Radiological appearances
1. There may be patchy areas of opacity scattered over the area which has been irradiated, or if the radiation dose is high, these areas may become confluent to produce an extensive area of consolidation (Figure 2.38a).
2. Complete resolution of the patchy changes may occur, but this is not usual with large areas of consolidation.
3. Large areas of consolidation usually progress to a coarse fibrosis and marked reduction in the volume of the area, resulting in displacement of moveable structures such as the hilar shadows, fissures and the mediastinum (Figure 2.38b).

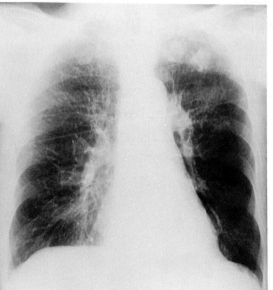

Fig. 2.38 (A) Acute radiation pneumonitis, left upper zone. (B) Chronic pulmonary radiation fibrosis, left upper zone. Note elevated left hilum.

SHOCK LUNG (ADULT RESPIRATORY DISTRESS SYNDROME)

In this condition, acute respiratory failure occurs in patients without major underlying lung disease. There is a large group of conditions which lead to the development of shock lung, such as extensive general body trauma, haemorrhagic or septic shock, acute pancreatitis, inhalation of gastric contents, traumatic fat embolism, and heroin or methadone overdose.

The changes which occur in the lung derive from an increased permeability of the capillaries and the alveolar epithelium. Conditions which may predispose to the changes are oxygen toxicity, left ventricular decompensation and prolonged respirator use.

Radiological appearances

1. No radiological changes are seen in the chest for approximately 12 hours after the onset of respiratory failure.

2. After 12 hours patchy, poorly defined areas of opacity appear in both lungs. These areas later coalesce to give massive consolidation of the lungs (Figure 2.39).

3. After approximately five days there is some clearing of the changes but the onset of acute pneumonia may produce localized areas of consolidation.

4. After some seven days a reticular pattern develops in the lung fields which is thought to be due to the development of pulmonary fibrosis.

Differential diagnosis

1. Pulmonary oedema of cardiac origin: usually the lungs are not so generally involved as in shock lung, but otherwise the appearances are very similar.

2. Inhalation of gastric contents: in this condition the radiological changes are immediate and not delayed as in other causes of shock lung.

3. Pulmonary contusion: the changes in the lungs are not delayed and usually clear reasonably rapidly.

4. Extensive pneumonia: distinguished only by clinical factors.

5. Massive thrombo-embolism: a lung scan will show evidence of the occluded vessels.

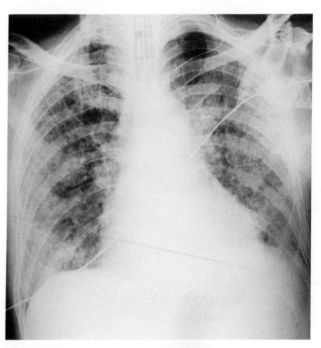

Fig. 2.39 'Shock lung', showing bilateral patchy consolidation.

TRAUMATIC FAT EMBOLISM

This condition usually follows fractures, particularly of large bones, and occurs one to two days after the trauma, which allows differentiation between this condition and pulmonary contusion. Resolution usually commences within a few days. The changes are due to globules of fat entering the circulation via torn veins and producing fat emboli in the lungs.

Radiological appearances

Scattered small areas of opacity with ill-defined margins in both lungs.

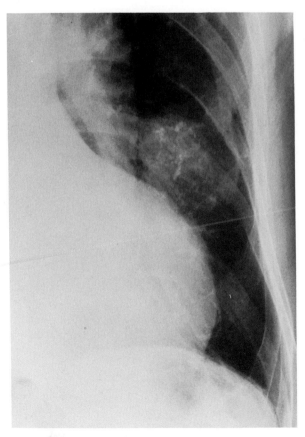

Fig. 2.40 Hamartoma, presenting as coin lesion, but showing characteristic 'pop-corn' calcification.

PULMONARY NEOPLASMS

Benign tumours

A number of benign tumours of the lung occur, but the commonest is the bronchial adenoma. All benign tumours are, however, rare by comparison with carcinoma of the bronchus, the ratio being of the order of 1:50

Bronchial adenoma

The most common site for adenomata is in large bronchi close to the hilum. The appearances depend on the size of the tumour. If small, the adenoma may occlude a bronchus and on a plain film only an area of collapsed lung is seen. A lung abscess may develop later in the area of collapse. If larger, the tumour itself may be seen as a sharply defined, lobulated, soft tissue opacity which may be discrete or fused with the hilar shadow. There may or may not be collapse of lung distal to the tumour. Adenomata which occur in the peripheral portion of the lung are seen as smooth, rounded, or lobulated opacities.

Pulmonary hamartoma

A hamartoma presents as a smooth, rounded or lobulated opacity roughly 2–4 cm in diameter. Calcification may be present in the mass and if the calcification resembles popcorn, the appearance is diagnostic (Figure 2.40).

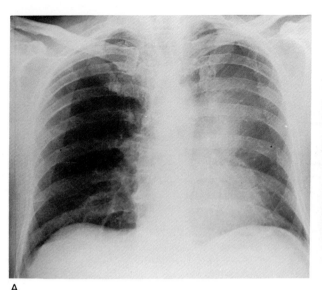
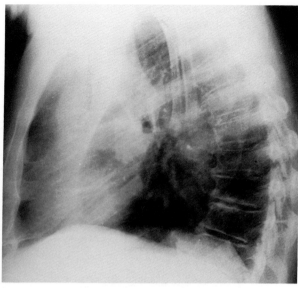

A   B

Fig. 2.41 Left bronchial carcinoma presenting as collapse of left upper lobe: (A) PA projection; (B) lateral projection.

Malignant tumours

Bronchogenic carcinoma
Carcinomata can be broadly divided into two types, those occurring centrally and those in the peripheral portion of the lung field. They are often associated with fluid in the pleural cavity.

Central tumour
The appearances depend on the size of the tumour and may present radiologically in five ways:

1. Bronchial obstruction. Collapse of a segment of lung or of a whole lobe may be all that is seen (Figure 2.41).

2. Unilateral enlarged or denser hilar shadow. This may result from the shadow of the tumour or of enlarged hilar nodes or a combination of both. A small tumour may produce a denser hilar shadow only. A large neoplasm will show enlargement of the hilar shadow with a 'hairy', ill-defined peripheral edge (Figure 2.42).

3. Bronchial obstruction plus enlarged hilum.

4. Widening of the mediastinum due to mediastinal node enlargement. There may be elevation of the diaphragm due to involvement of the phrenic nerve by enlarged nodes.

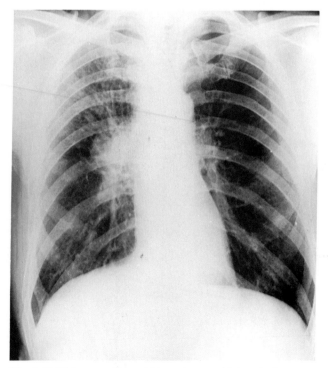

Fig. 2.42 Right central bronchial carcinoma with lymphatic spread to right upper lobe.

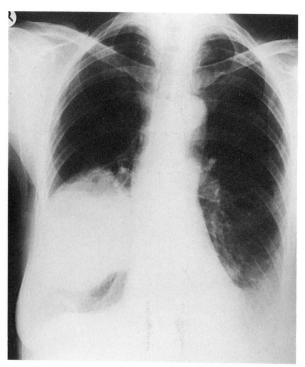

Fig. 2.43 Large right basal peripheral lung carcinoma.

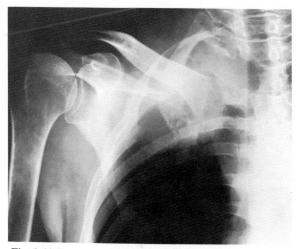

Fig. 2.44 Pancoast tumour of lung apex, with rib destruction.

5. Slow or incomplete resolution of pneumonia. Infection with consolidation may occur distal to a broncho-stenotic lesion; the area of opacity clears slowly and incompletely on standard therapy. Enlarged hilar nodes may be present (compare simple pneumonia, page 30).

Peripheral tumour
Peripheral carcinomata present radiologically in one of three ways:

1. A localized, fairly well-defined, rounded area of opacity in the peripheral portion of the lung field, which can vary in size from less than 1 cm in diameter up to a large mass. There may be a dimple-like depression in the margin (umbilication). There may be linear strands connecting it to the hilum and these are due to congested lymphatics.

2. Single or multiple areas of opacity, which may be bilateral and which have irregular, ill-defined edges (Figure 2.43).

3. The superior sulcus or Pancoast tumour. It presents as an area of uniform opacity at the apex of the lung, and is associated with localized destruction of ribs and involvement of the sympathetic chain to produce Horner's syndrome (Figure 2.44).

There is a tendency for peripheral carcinomata to undergo central necrosis and cavitation. The cavity as seen on the radiograph usually has a thick wall which is irregular on its inner surface. There may be necrotic material lying in the cavity and the appearances are then difficult to differentiate from those of a mycetoma.

Computerized tomography is particularly useful to delineate the location, extent, and spread of a carcinoma, as well as showing whether hilar and mediastinal nodes are involved.

COIN LESIONS
Coin lesion is the name given to a small, round opacity in the lung field. There are a great number of conditions which produce such a lesion, but the four most common by far are primary carcinoma, granuloma, hamartoma and metastasis.

Differential diagnosis

There are certain general points which help in the differentiation of these conditions. Carcinoma is much more common in males than in females, and over the age of 40 carcinoma becomes more common and granuloma less common. Tomography is the best method of examination of the edge and contents of the nodule.

1. Carcinoma: the margin is usually ill-defined and the nodule may show umbilication. Carcinomata almost never calcify so that the presence of calcification within the lesion virtually excludes carcinoma. Satellite lesions may be present.

2. Granuloma: tuberculoma would be the most common granuloma seen, except in certain parts of America where histoplasmosis and coccidiomycosis are more common. Calcification is common and craggy in nature. The margin of the nodule is usually ill-defined. There may be cavitation present and satellite lesions are common.

3. Hamartoma: these nodules are sharply defined and often contain calcified areas. Sometimes the calcification resembles 'popcorn' and this appearance is diagnostic (see Figure 2.40). There are no satellite lesions.

4. Metastasis: these are sharply defined and round. Calcification is very rare although metastases from an osteogenic sarcoma may produce bone. Cavitation is rarely seen. Satellite lesions do not occur.

HYDATID

Although it is not a neoplasm it presents as a mass and is most conveniently dealt with here. Hydatid of the lung presents as a round, sharply defined opacity and may be single or multiple (Figure 2.45). Lung hydatids never calcify but they may rupture and, with discharge of the contents, a cavity may be left which may form the site of a mycetoma. Sometimes after rupture the inner lining may collapse and lie on the surface of fluid in the cavity giving the appearance of a water-lily floating on the fluid (Figure 2.46).

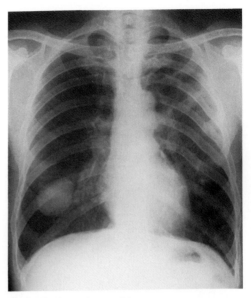

Fig. 2.45 Hydatid cyst of lung.

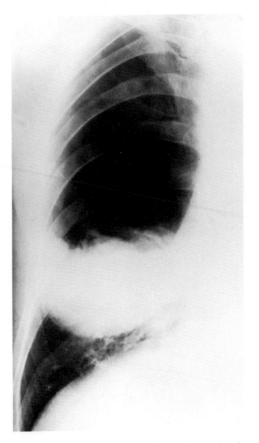

Fig. 2.46 Ruptured right basal hydatid cyst showing the 'waterlily sign'.

HODGKIN'S DISEASE

In the vast majority of cases (90%) the chest is involved in the changes of Hodgkin's disease. The mediastinal lymph nodes and the lungs may both be involved, but involvement of the lymph nodes alone is considerably more common.

Radiological appearances

1. Mediastinal lymph nodes: there is enlargement of lymph nodes, particularly in the paratracheal area, but enlargement of nodes at the hila, the retrosternal area and carina is also common (Figure 2.47a). The enlargement tends to be asymmetrical and bilateral and results in: (a) broadening of the upper mediastinal shadow, which may also have a lobulated margin; (b) well-defined enlargement of the hilar shadows which are also often lobulated; (c) obliteration of the retrosternal window by enlargement of the thymus and nodes. This helps to distinguish the appearances from sarcoidosis in which the retrosternal nodes are seldom involved (Figure 2.47b).

Computerized tomography is the examination of choice to show mediastinal involvement.

2. Lung changes. There are two main patterns within the lungs: (a) linear and nodular areas of opacity extending out into the lung fields from the hila; (b) areas of consolidation in the lung field which may coalesce to form large areas of opacity. Occasionally there is a miliary nodulation present. Cavitation may occur within

A
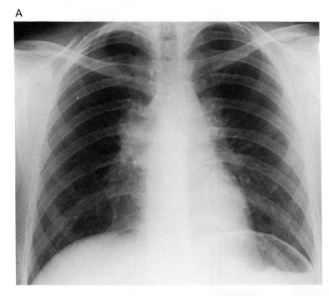

Fig. 2.47 Hodgkins disease producing lymph node enlargement.
(A) PA radiograph showing enlarged hilar nodes.
(B) Lateral radiograph showing enlarged retrosternal nodes (→).
(C) CT scan of chest, showing enlarged anterior mediastinal lymph nodes.

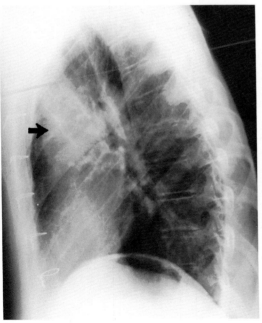

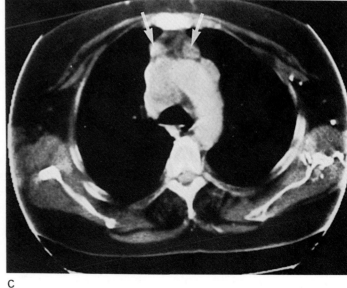

C

B

the areas of lung consolidation and Kerley B lines resulting from lymphatic obstruction are common (see page 49).

3. Pleura and pericardium: involvement of the pleura and pericardium may lead to pleural or pericardial effusions.

Differential diagnosis

1. Carcinoma of the bronchus: this tends to occur in an older age group.

2. Tuberculous cavitation: secondary tuberculosis does not have mediastinal node enlargement.

3. Sarcoidosis: when the lung changes are of a miliary character or only mediastinal nodes are involved radiological differentiation may not be possible. Enlarged retrosternal nodes suggest Hodgkin's disease rather than sarcoidosis.

SARCOIDOSIS

Although sarcoidosis can affect many organs, the lungs and hilar nodes are the most common sites of involvement. A significant factor in the diagnosis is the presence of gross changes on the chest radiograph in a patient who is clinically showing little evidence of ill health. Radiologically there may be changes in the mediastinal lymph glands alone or in combination with lung changes, or there may be lung changes alone.

Radiological appearances

1. **Nodes**: there is enlargement of mediastinal nodes, particularly those at the hila and to a lesser extent in the paratracheal area (Figure 2.48). Retrosternal nodes are rarely involved (compare Hodgkin's disease). The hilar shadows are therefore enlarged, sharply defined and often lobulated. The hilar enlargement is symmetrical and bilateral. The nodes rarely calcify but if they do the calcification occurs in a rim around the edge of the node — 'egg-shell calcification'.

2. **Lung**.

   (a) Nodules: there may be a miliary nodulation throughout both lung fields. The nodules may be very small, as in miliary tuberculosis, or up to 5 mm in diameter (Figure 2.49).

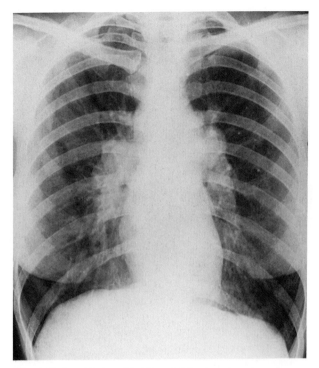

Fig. 2.48 Sarcoidosis, with bilateral hilar lymph node enlargement.

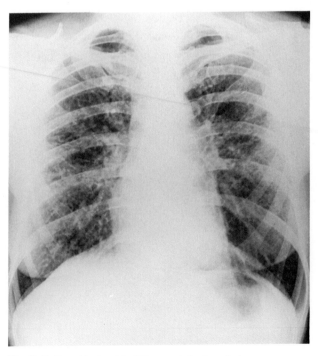

Fig. 2.49 Sarcoidosis with diffuse nodular lung lesions.

(b) Coarse lung pattern: there may be a
fine or a coarse network of abnormal
markings present throughout both
lungs. This may occur in association
with the miliary nodulation.

(c) Localized opacities: round opacities
very similar in appearance to metastases
may be scattered throughout the lungs,
or the opacities may have ill-defined
edges and resemble areas of
inflammatory changes. These opacities
never calcify (compare tuberculosis),
but may rarely cavitate.

(d) Pulmonary fibrosis: although the
changes in the lungs and nodes may
persist for a long period, up to two
years, complete resolution of all
changes is the result in the majority
(80%) of cases. In the remaining cases
coarse, irregular, linear strands of
fibrous tissue develop, radiating out
from the hila into the lung fields.
There is a tendency for the upper
portions of the lungs to be involved
more than the lower zones, and
elevation of the hilar shadows due to
the contraction of the fibrous tissue is
common (Figure 2.50). Emphysematous
changes occur between the areas of
fibrosis and eventually there may be
evidence of pulmonary hypertension
and cor pulmonale.

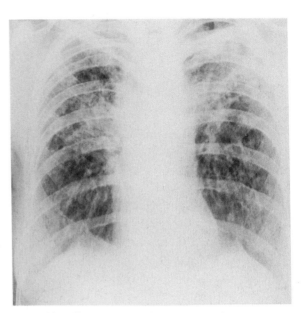

Fig. 2.50 Diffuse pulmonary fibrosis due to chronic
sarcoidosis.

Differential diagnosis
The main condition to be distinguished from
sarcoidosis is Hodgkin's disease. The following
points are helpful:

1. Hodgkin's disease tends to affect the
paratracheal nodes more than the hilar nodes. In
sarcoidosis the hilar nodes are predominantly
affected.

2. Node enlargement in Hodgkin's disease
tends to be asymmetrical, but symmetrical in
sarcoidosis.

3. Retrosternal node enlargement is common
in Hodgkin's disease and rare in sarcoidosis.

EMPHYSEMA

Radiologically there are three main types of pulmonary emphysema:

1. Primary emphysema
2. Obstructive emphysema
3. Compensatory emphysema.

It is important to remember that primary emphysematous changes must be well advanced before radiological signs become manifest.

Primary emphysema

Radiological appearances (Figure 2.51)

1. Diminution in the size and number of vascular markings: this is the most important criterion in the diagnosis of emphysema and is best seen in the peripheral portions of the lung fields.

2. Enlarged hilar shadows: this is frequently seen and is due to dilatation of the main pulmonary arteries.

3. Hypertranslucent lung fields.

4. Depressed diaphragm: the domes of the diaphragm are usually depressed to or beyond the llth rib in inspiration. There is also reduced excursion of the diaphragm, which normally moves about two intercostal spaces with respiration.

5. Enlarged retrosternal window: this window is increased in width and extends down further in front of the heart than normal.

6. Long, thin heart shadow: this results from depression of the diaphgram and consequent rotation of the heart.

7. Bullae: these are localized, round, air-containing cystic spaces with very thin walls. They vary in size from less than 1 cm in diameter to large cysts which can occupy most of the lung. They are best seen along the margins of the lung.

8. Skeletal changes: there is often a fairly marked kyphosis of the dorsal spine and forward bowing of the sternum.

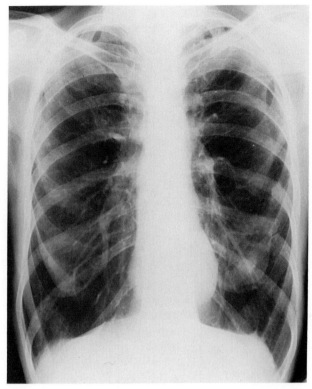

Fig. 2.51 Emphysema with overinflated lungs, and depressed diaphragms.

Obstructive emphysema

This occurs distal to a ball-valve obstruction of a bronchus, which allows air to pass during inspiration but prevents escape of air on expiration. It is seen most commonly in children with an inhaled foreign body (Figure 2.52) and sometimes in adults with a bronchial carcinoma. The area of emphysema will depend on the size of the bronchus which is blocked.

Compensatory emphysema

When one portion of the lung collapses or is reduced in volume by fibrosis, there is often some shift of the mediastinal shadows to the affected side; in addition the remainder of the lung undergoes hyperexpansion to take up the space normally occupied by the affected portion of the lung. If a whole lung is affected, compensatory emphysema will be apparent in the opposite lung.

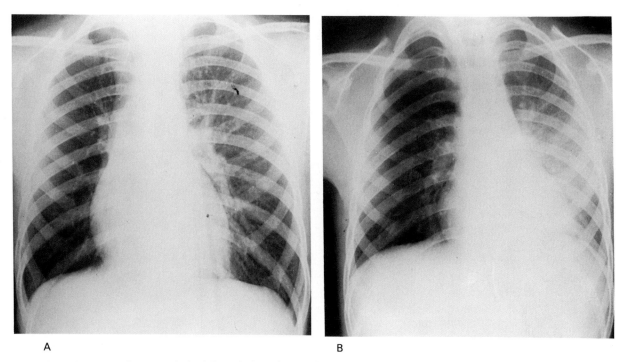

A   B

Fig. 2.52 Inhaled foreign body in right main bronchus producing air trapping.
A. Inspiratory radiograph appears normal. B. Expiratory radiograph shows relative overexpansion of right lung.

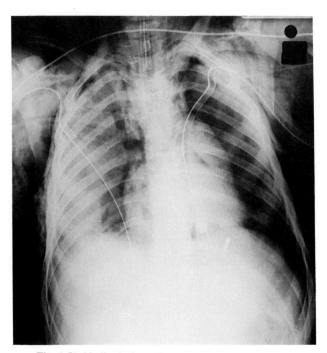

Fig. 2.53 Mediastinal emphysema.

MEDIASTINAL EMPHYSEMA

This term is applied to the presence of free air in the mediastinum. It appears as irregular linear areas of translucency and may outline the margin of the heart shadow as a dark line due to separation of the pleura from the mediastinum by the air (Figure 2.53). It may be seen in the following circumstances:
1. Penetrating wound
2. Perforation of the oesophagus or trachea
3. Asthma and whooping cough
4. New born infants
5. Lacerated lung.

Except in infants, when it tends to be confined to the mediastinum, the air may extend up into the neck and produce subcutaneous emphysema, which shows as areas of translucency in the soft tissues.

ASTHMA

Radiological appearances

1. The appearances on the radiograph may be normal.

2. During an attack of asthma there may be (a) normal appearances, and (b) hyperinflation of the lungs which shows as increased translucency of the lung fields, but in contrast with emphysema the lung markings in the peripheral portions of the lung fields are normal although more spread out. Hyperinflation produces depression of the diaphragm and reduced excursion of this structure.

In addition to the above changes, there are a number of less common changes which can occur.

1. Mediastinal emphysema: following rupture of alveoli, air escapes along the interstitial spaces of the lung to reach the mediastinum, where it can be seen as a thin black line outlining the mediastinal shadow.

2. Pneumothorax: due to rupture of alveoli or bullae.

3. Areas of consolidation: these are transient and tend to appear and disappear in different parts of the lung. It is considered that they are due to hypersensitivity reactions to pulmonary aspergillosis.

4. Areas of collapse: these may be large or small and are probably due to obstruction of bronchi by mucus plugs.

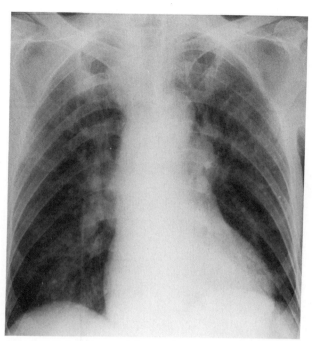

Fig. 2.54 Enlarged upper lobe vessels due to blood diversion in heart failure.

CONGESTIVE CARDIAC FAILURE AND PULMONARY OEDEMA

The most common cause of raised pulmonary venous pressure is left heart failure, which may arise from a variety of causes such as aortic or mitral valvular disease, systemic hypertension, or myocardial infarction. This gives rise to a back-up of blood in the pulmonary venous circulation and hence a rise in venous pressure.

Radiological appearances

The earliest signs of this condition are dilatation of the veins running from the hilum to the apex of the lung (Figure 2.54) and Kerley B lines.

Kerley B lines are short, white, linear shadows which run for a short distance transversely across the lung at the base from the pleural surface and are due to congested interlobular lymphatics or oedematous interlobular septa (Figure 2.55). Kerley B lines may be seen in a variety of conditions:

1. Left heart failure
2. Obstruction of lymphatic flow: (a) silicosis; (b) malignant obstruction of lymphatics or malignant involvement of hilar glands; (c) sarcoidosis.

As the pressure in the pulmonary veins increases, fluid collects in the interstitial spaces in the lungs — interstitial oedema — and results in haziness of the vascular markings and of the hilar shadows on the radiograph.

As the condition progresses fluid commences to accumulate in the alveoli also — air space oedema — and poorly defined patches of opacity appear in the lung fields. These areas may become confluent to produce widespread opacity within which may be seen an air-bronchogram. In some cases the areas of opacity are peri-hilar, sparing the peripheral portion of the lungs to produce the 'bat's wing' appearance (Figure 2.56). Pulmonary oedema is usually bilateral and symmetrical but may be unilateral. It may also be seen in conditions other than cardiac failure such as following the inhalation of irritant gases or regurgitated and inhaled gastric contents.

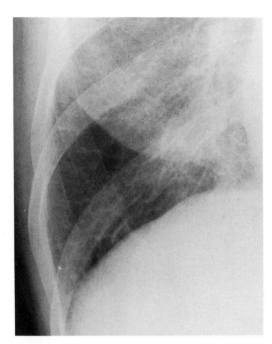

Fig. 2.55 Kerley B lines, due to septal lymphatic engorgement, usually in heart failure.

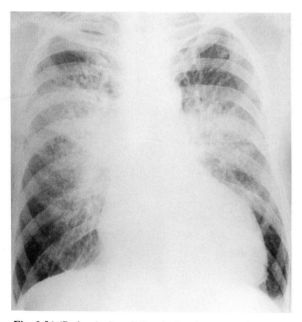

Fig. 2.56 'Bat's wing' perihilar shadow in acute pulmonary oedema.

PULMONARY EMBOLISM

Embolism is a relatively common and potentially lethal cause of dyspnoea, pleuritic pain, and occasionally haemoptysis.

Radiological appearances

1. Chest radiographs are usually normal although a small effusion may be present. If infarction has occurred it will produce one or more localized opacities extending to the pleura and indistinguishable from a small area of inflammation or collapse.

2. Radionuclide perfusion scanning with intravenous labelled particles will show pulmonary artery blood flow distribution. An occluded segment will not contain activity (Figure 2.57a). Other causes of maldistribution include emphysema, asthma, bronchitis, pneumonia, neoplasms, or any other cause of segmentally reduced ventilation.

Differentiation is partly by chest radiography and partly by a radionuclide ventilation scan.

3. Radionuclide ventilation scans show the transit of gas (usually ^{133}Xe) to the various segments of the lungs. Disparity between ventilation and perfusion distribution is required to diagnose embolism (Figure 2.57b).

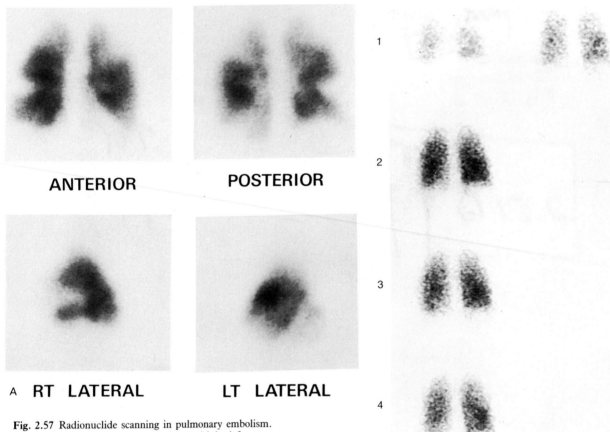

ANTERIOR   POSTERIOR

A RT LATERAL   LT LATERAL

1

2

3

4

B

Fig. 2.57 Radionuclide scanning in pulmonary embolism.
(A) Perfusion scan showing multiple defects.
(B) Ventilation scan essentially normal.

4. Pulmonary angiography (Figure 2.58). The 'gold standard' for the detection of embolism is the pulmonary angiogram. This is usually performed by the passage of a venous catheter into the pulmonary arteries via the right heart, and injection of contrast medium producing images of arteries and veins. The recent development of digital subtraction angiography enables pulmonary angiography to be performed by injection into a peripheral vein using much smaller quantities of contrast medium (see (page 5).

Diagnostic decision tree 1, page 300, gives a suggested sequence of investigations for suspected pulmonary embolism.

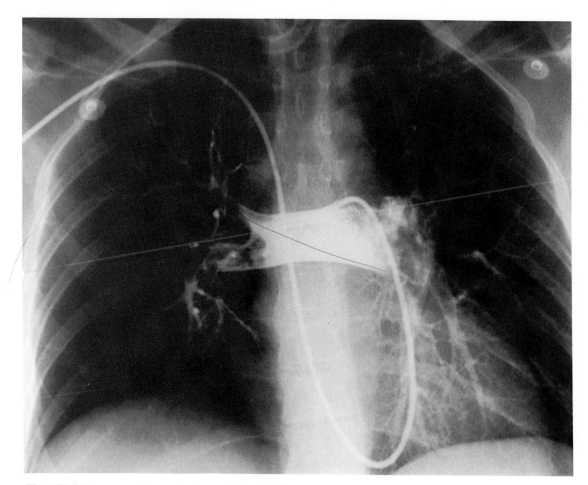

Fig. 2.58 Pulmonary angiogram showing multiple emboli.

INORGANIC DUST DISEASES

Silicosis

Silicosis results from the inhalation of silica or silicon dioxide particles over a long period. A number of occupations are involved including quartz mining and sand blasting.

Radiological appearances

1. Reticular pattern: this is often the earliest sign and consists of a network of linear shadows throughout the lungs.

2. Nodules: multiple well-defined nodules up to 10 mm in diameter appear in the medial portions of the mid and upper zones of the lungs, and later spread to involve the remainder of the lungs although to a lesser degree (Figure 2.59a).

3. Hilar lymph nodes: enlargement of these nodes is common and they may show a rim of calcification — 'egg-shell calcification' — or be uniformly calcified (Figure 2.59b). Egg-shell calcification is almost diagnostic of silicosis although it does occasionally occur in sarcoidosis.

4. Consolidation: late in the disease the nodules in the lungs may coalesce and produce areas of consolidation with ill-defined margins in the upper portions of the lungs. The remainder of the lungs become emphysematous and there is evidence of fibrosis in the lung fields (Figure 2.59c).

5. Cavitation: silicosis predisposes to tuberculosis and the changes of tuberculous infection including cavitation may appear at the apices.

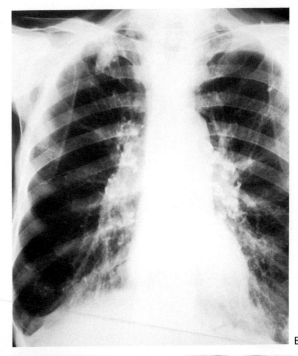

B

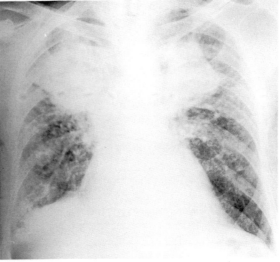

C

A

Fig. 2.59 (A) Nodular stage of silicosis.
  (B) Silicosis with calcified hilar lymph nodes.
  (C) Silicosis with bilateral progressive massive fibrosis.

Asbestosis

Asbestosis occurs most frequently in miners but may also occur in persons using asbestos industrially (Figure 2.60).

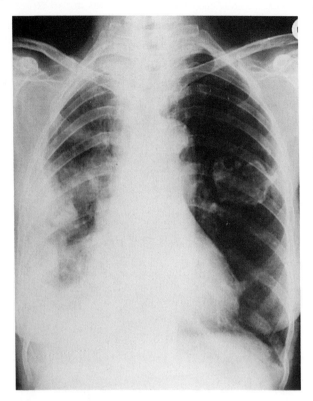

Fig. 2.60 Asbestosis with pleural calcifications and a right basal mesothelioma.

ORGANIC DUST DISEASES

The changes which occur in the lungs result from a hypersensitivity to the inhaled material and occur in such conditions as bagassosis (sugar cane processing), byssinosis (cotton cleaning), pigeon breeders' lung, malt workers' lung, farmers' lung, and many others.

Radiological appearances

In general, these conditions show a fine nodulation throughout the lungs which is often associated with a network of linear markings. There may also be larger areas of opacity present in the acute stage.

Radiological appearances

1. Fibrosis: bilateral interstitial fibrosis, characterized by an increase in linear markings and shrinkage of the areas of lung involved, develops in the lower portions of the lungs and may later spread throughout the lungs. This is the first sign of the disease.

2. Shaggy heart: the cardiac outline often becomes ill-defined and shaggy due to adhesions.

3. Pleural changes: areas of thickened pleura are common and plaques of calcification may occur within these areas.

4. Neoplastic changes: asbestosis predisposes to the development of bronchial carcinoma and pleural mesothelioma, and changes due to these conditions may be added to the general picture.

THE CHEST IN PAEDIATRICS

NEONATAL RESPIRATORY DISTRESS SYNDROME

There are a number of conditions which may cause respiratory distress in the newborn, but only those which are relatively common are dealt with here. For a complete survey of the causes the reader is referred to paediatric radiology texts.

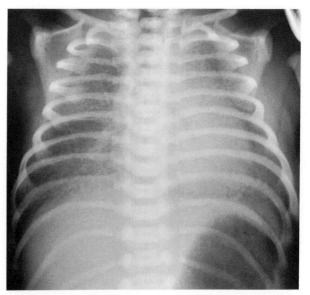

Fig. 2.61 Hyaline membrane disease in a premature neonate. Note the ground-glass appearance, and air bronchogram.

Hyaline membrane disease

This condition is prone to occur in premature infants, particularly if they have suffered from anoxia. The changes in the lungs usually develop within several hours of birth and are well established by 12 hours. They consist of fine miliary nodulation in the lung fields which may be uniformly distributed throughout both lungs or be more marked in the lower zones (Figure 2.61) and may produce a ground glass appearance. Occasionally only one lung or part of one lung is affected. The nodulation is accompanied by an air bronchogram. These changes may commence clearing or become much more marked over the ensuing few days. There may be evidence of associated cardiac enlargement.

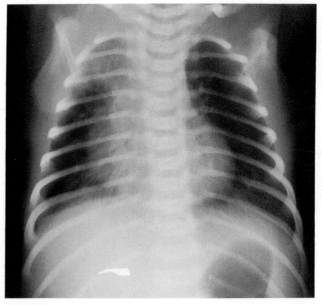

Fig. 2.62 Neonatal lung atelectasis, affecting right upper lobe, and to a lesser extent the lung bases.

Atelectasis

This condition tends to occur more frequently in premature infants and may involve both lungs, or the whole or part of one lung. The changes are present at birth. There is uniform opacity of the involved area, and an air bronchogram is present (Figure 2.62). If it is unilateral there may be shift of the mediastinal structures towards the affected side.

Pneumothorax

The edge of the partially collapsed lung can be seen and, if there is a tension pneumothorax present, displacement of the mediastinal structures away from the side of the pneumothorax occurs. When a tension pneumothorax is present there may not necessarily be complete collapse of the lung on the affected side.

Congenital cystic lung

The lung is opaque and contains well-defined translucent cystic areas. The mediastinum is usually displaced away from the involved lung.

Cystic fibrosis (mucoviscidosis)

In this condition the mucus in the bronchi is more viscid than normal and causes bronchial obstruction which may be followed by infection in the obstructed area. This may lead on to the development of bronchiectasis. As the result of the obstruction there may be either collapse or hyperinflation of the lung area involved. Recurrent areas of pneumonic change develop in the area, and these may lead to abscess formation or thin-walled cysts similar to those seen in staphylococcal pneumonia (Figure 2.63).

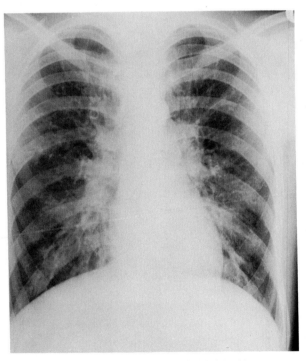

Fig. 2.63 Fibrocystic disease (mucoviscidosis) with bronchiectasis and peribronchial consolidation.

Diaphragmatic hernia

There is an area of opacity, within which there may be seen gas containing loops of bowel, in the hemithorax.

The mediastinal shadow may be displaced away from this area.

INHALED FOREIGN BODY

The foreign body may be seen if radio-opaque. Distal to the foreign body there may be pulmonary collapse showing as an area of opacity, or if the foreign body acts in a ball-valve fashion there may be hyperinflation of the involved area of lung (see obstructive emphysema, page 46). Films of the chest made on inspiration and expiration may show a persistent area of radiolucency in part of the lung due to the presence of air trapped beyond a foreign body which is obstructing a branch bronchus (see Figure 2.52).

VARICELLA (CHICKEN POX) PNEUMONIA

There is a widespread nodularity in the lungs and with healing some of these nodules may calcify to give scattered small areas of calcification in the lungs (Figure 2.64).

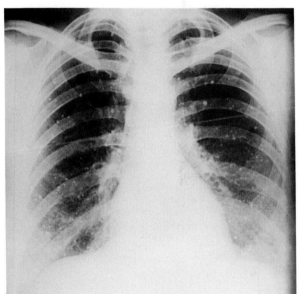

Fig. 2.64 Multiple small calcified lung opacities from previous varicella pneumonia.

THYMIC ENLARGEMENT

Enlargement of the thymus, showing as a triangular 'sail-shaped' opacity adjacent to the right side of the mediastinum just above the hilum, is sometimes seen in infants and should not be confused with an area of consolidation or collapse of the lung (see Figure 3.34).

MEDIASTINAL MASSES

A high percentage of mediastinal masses are symptomless and are found only when a chest radiograph is made for some reason such as a pre-operative chest examination.

Broadly speaking, there are three compartments in the mediastinum: the anterior compartment between heart and sternum; the posterior compartment between heart and thoracic spine; and the central compartment containing the heart, great vessels, trachea and lung roots.

The most important radiological point to establish is the compartment of the mediastinum in which the lesion lies, because although there is some overlap the different types of masses tend to occur predominantly in certain compartments (Figure 2.65).

Computerized tomography is the examination of choice, defining the site and extent of the lesion, and often indicating its nature by the internal tissue characteristics.

ANTERIOR MEDIASTINAL MASSES
The following masses occur in the anterior mediastinum (Figure 2.65):
1. Retrosternal thyroid mass
2. Thymoma
3. Teratomas and dermoid cysts
4. Enlarged lymph nodes
5. Lipoma
6. Pericardial cyst
7. Diaphragmatic hernia.

It is frequently impossible to differentiate radiologically between these conditions. They may all present simply as a well-defined rounded opacity and several may on occasion be lobulated. The following features may, however, assist in reaching a reasonably accurate decision on the nature of a mass.

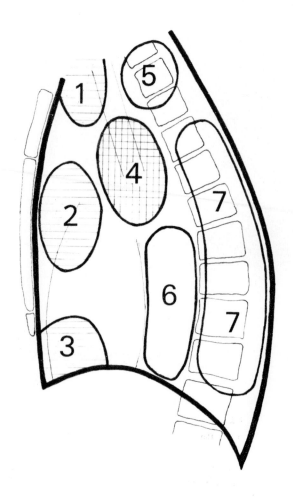

Fig. 2.65 (Sutton) Typical sites of common mediastinal masses:

Anterior division	1. Lymph node enlargement Retrosternal thyroid mass
	2. Lymph node enlargement Aneurysm of ascending aorta Thymoma Terato–dermoid tumour Lipoma
	3. Fat-pad Foramen of Morgagani hernia Pericardial cyst Diaphragmatic hump
Middle division	4. Enlarged lymph nodes Aneurysm of aortic arch Bronchogenic cyst Enlarged pulmonary artery
Posterior division	5. Pharyngeal pouch Neurogenic tumour
	6. Hiatus hernia Dilated oesophagus Aneurysm of the descending aorta
	7. Foramen of Bochdalek hernia Neurogenic tumour Para-vertebral mass

Retrosternal thyroid masses

They are usually symptomless and may be rounded or lobulated. They are most commonly situated in the upper part of the anterior compartment from where they may be seen to extend up into the neck, although they may also occur in the posterior compartment.

Nodular calcification is often present in the mass. If active thyroid tissue is present in the mass, which is rare, radionuclide studies may give the diagnosis.

Thymoma

Approximately 50% are associated with myasthenia gravis. They are usually rounded but may be lobulated and occur most commonly behind the manubrium sterni. Calcification may be present, scattered throughout the tumour (Figure 2.66 and see Figure 3.35).

Teratomas and dermoid cysts

These occur most commonly behind the body of the sternum and are usually symptomless. They are usually rounded but a malignant teratoma may be lobulated. Calcification may be scattered throughout the mass and if fat is present it may produce areas of radiolucency within the tumour. The presence of a tooth or of bone within the mass is diagnostic.

Enlarged lymph nodes

These may be due to lymphomas, leukaemia, metastases, or granulomas and may thus be associated with signs and symptoms of these conditions. The most common site is in the region of the internal mammary arteries behind the body of the sternum. They may be smoothly rounded or lobulated. Calcification may be present in the mass if it is due to a granuloma.

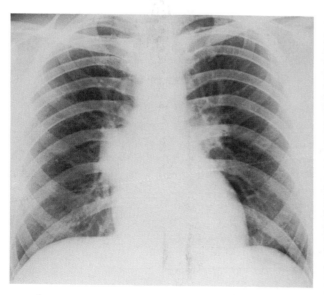

A

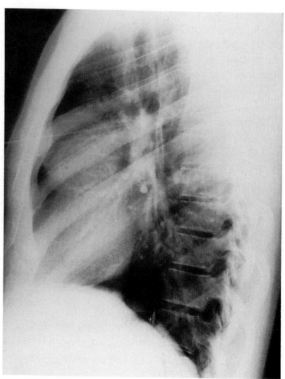

B

Fig. 2.66 Thymoma shown to lie in anterior mediastinum on PA (A) and lateral (B) chest radiographs.

Lipoma
These are symptomless. They may be relatively radiolucent for the size of the mass, or opaque. They are commonly lobulated.

Pericardial cysts
These are usually symptomless and tend to be rounded but may change shape with changes in posture or with respiration. The most common site is in the angle between the diaphragm and the sternum on the right side.

Diaphragmatic herniae
These are almost invariably symptomless. Herniation of abdominal contents occurs through the foramen of Morgagni and the mass is thus situated in the angle between the sternum and diaphragm anteriorly. The mass is rounded and smooth. The mass may be uniformly opaque or if it contains bowel, gas shadows may be visible.

POSTERIOR MEDIASTINAL MASSES
The most common posterior mediastinal masses (Figure 2.65) are:
1. Neurogenic tumours
2. Neuroenteric cysts
3. Oesophageal abnormalities
4. Diaphragmatic hernia
5. Thoracic spine abnormalities.

The majority of posterior mediastinal masses are symptomless and they may all present as well-defined, rounded opacities. The following features may help in differentiating between the various masses.

Neurogenic tumours
It is usually not possible to differentiate radiologically between the various types of neurogenic tumours, but neuroblastomas tend to occur in young children while other neurogenic tumours have a peak incidence in young adults.

They are situated in the paravertebral region (Figure 2.67) and some are associated with spinal abnormalities. Some give rise to erosion of ribs and vertebrae, and dumb-bell tumours (partly inside the spinal canal and partly outside) may cause enlargement of a neural foramen.

Neurogenic tumours are usually rounded. Lobulation does not occur.

Neurenteric cysts
These are usually painful and form rounded, masses. They may contain gas (if there is a patent connection with the oesophagus or upper gastrointestinal tract). They are often associated with congenital defects of the thoracic spine.

Oesophageal abnormalities
1. Oesophageal tumours: carcinoma of the oesophagus is rarely large enough to present as a mass on the chest radiograph, but benign tumours such as leiomyoma are often large and present as a rounded mass. A contrast swallow may indicate its nature.
2. Hiatus hernia: this may be seen as a rounded mass just above the diaphragm and behind the heart. There may be a fluid level within the mass.
3. Dilated oesophagus: there are several causes such as achalasia, benign stricture and carcinoma. It appears as a mottled shadow behind the heart and usually has a fluid level at the upper end.

Diaphragmatic hernia
This occurs in the posterior costophrenic angle, where the contents protrude through the foramen of Bochdalek. The hernia is well defined, rounded and opaque, and is found most commonly in children.

Thoracic spine abnormalities
Tuberculous infections may be associated with a spindle-shaped mass around dorsal vertebrae, which show disc narrowing and bone erosion.

Neoplasms rarely produce a significant mass but enlargement of nodes in Hodgkin's disease may produce a paravertebral spindle-shaped mass. There may be other evidence of Hodgkin's disease on clinical examination.

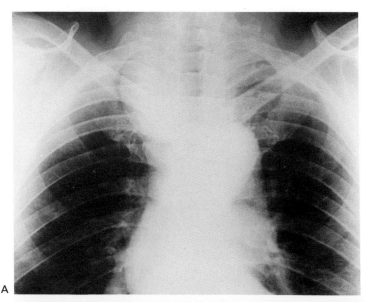
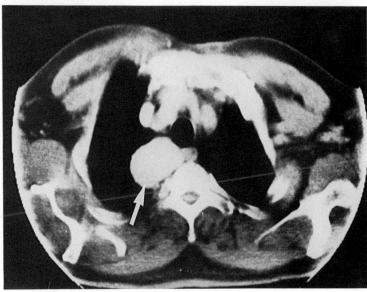

Fig. 2.67 Neurofibroma.
(A) Mass at right apex on chest radiograph.
(B) CT scan shows the mass to be paravertebral, and solid. No intracanalicular extension is seen.

MIDDLE MEDIASTINAL MASSES
The most common middle mediastinal masses are:
1. Lymph node enlargement
2. Aortic arch aneurysm
3. Bronchogenic cyst.

Lymph node enlargement
This is the most common cause of a mediastinal mass and may result from lymphomata,

reticuloses, leukaemia, metastases, sarcoidosis or primary tuberculosis.

1. Hodgkin's disease and leukaemia: the paratracheal nodes are most commonly involved and cause a widening of the upper mediastinal shadow, which usually has a lobulated margin. If the hilar nodes are involved, the hilar shadows are enlarged and usually lobulated.

2. Metastatic carcinoma: the hilar nodes are nearly always involved to give enlargement and

lobulation of the hilar shadows. In carcinoma of
the lung the node enlargement is most
commonly unilateral.

3. Sarcoidosis: the hilar nodes are the most
commonly affected and the changes are usually
bilateral and symmetrical, so that both hilar
shadows show a lobulated enlargement. Less
commonly, the paratracheal nodes are enlarged
and these may cause widening of the upper
mediastinal shadow with lobulation of the
margin. It is frequently associated with bilateral
lung changes, particularly of a miliary type.

4. Tuberculosis: hilar and sometimes
paratracheal node enlargement is seen in *primary*
tuberculosis. It is seen as enlargement of the
hilum or widening of the mediastinal shadow.

The node enlargement is usually unilateral, and
craggy calcification may later develop in the
nodes.

Aortic arch aneurysm
This produces a fusiform or rounded shadow in
the line of the aorta and may have a calcified
margin. The mass may be seen to be pulsatile
on fluoroscopy but it is often non-pulsatile.
Aortography produces a definite diagnosis.

Bronchogenic cyst
Usually symptomless, it tends to occur in young
people. It produces a round, well-defined opacity
in the region of the carina and may project out
beyond the hilum in the postero-anterior
radiograph.

The paranasal sinuses

METHODS OF INVESTIGATION

Plain radiographs
These are the most common method of
investigating sinus pathology.

Tomography
Blowout fractures of the orbit involve the roof of
the maxillary antrum or the lateral wall of the
ethmoid cells and are better demonstrated by
tomography than by plain films.

Computerized tomography
This may show blowout fractures and other
sinus pathology more clearly and more reliably
than plain tomograms.

TRAUMATIC LESIONS
Involvement of the paranasal sinuses by facial
fractures is described in the section on skull
fractures. Blow out fractures of the orbit may
show a fracture of the roof of the antrum or
opacity of the ethmoid cells (see Figure 6.14).

INFLAMMATION AND ALLERGY
These conditions both produce swelling of the
lining mucosa of sinuses and both may be
responsible for a collection of fluid in a sinus.
Mucosal swelling may be seen as an opaque
layer around the inner margin of the frontal
sinuses or antra (Figure 2.68) and if this layer is
lobulated it is more suggestive of allergic than of
inflammatory change (Figure 2.69). The mucosal

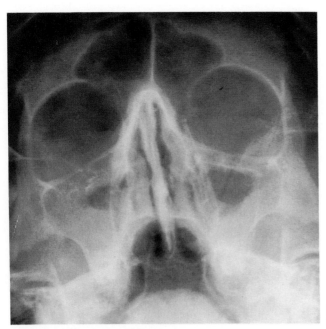

Fig. 2.68 Generalized mucosal thickening in the paranasal sinuses.

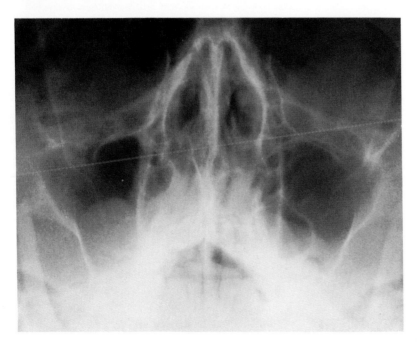

Fig. 2.69 Mucosal polyp on floor of right maxillary antrum.

swelling may, however, be so gross that it fills the sinus cavity and the sinus is then uniformly opaque.

Mucosal swelling in the ethmoid cells renders them opaque.

If there is only a small or moderate amount of fluid present in a sinus a fluid level will be seen (Figure 2.70), but if there is a large collection the sinus will be uniformly opaque.

The differential diagnosis between allergic and inflammatory changes usually depends on the clinical findings. Occasionally inflammatory lesions in the sinuses, particularly the frontal sinuses, may involve the surrounding bone to produce an osteomyelitis. The frontal sinus has a sharply defined, thin, dense, bony margin, but with the onset of osteomyelitis there is loss of definition of the margin, patchy osteoporosis in the adjacent bone, and opacity of the sinus. As with osteomyelitis in other bones, the clinical signs and symptoms precede the radiological evidence by several days.

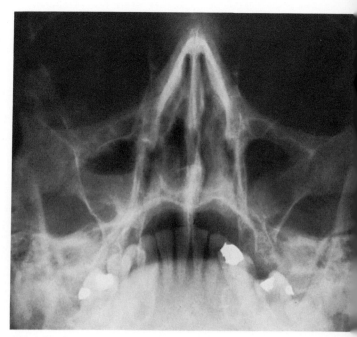

Fig. 2.70 Fluid level in right maxillary antrum in case of acute infective sinusitis.

NEOPLASMS

Osteoma
This is the most common benign tumour and may be a very dense, ivory osteoma (Figure 2.71) or very poorly calcified. They are most common in the frontal sinuses.

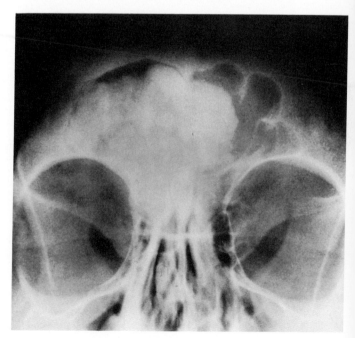

Fig. 2.71 Large ivory osteoma of frontal sinus.

Carcinoma

This is by far the most common malignant tumour in the paranasal sinuses and occurs most frequently in the maxillary antrum or the ethmoid sinuses.

   1. plain films: (a) opacity of the sinus; (b) destruction of the bony wall of the sinus.

   2. Computerized tomography: this is especially useful in demonstrating destruction of the bony walls of sinuses and the spread of a tumour into adjacent soft tissues (Figure 2.72).

Fig. 2.72 CT scan showing carcinoma of left ethmoidal sinuses with spread to sphenoid sinus, and bone destruction.

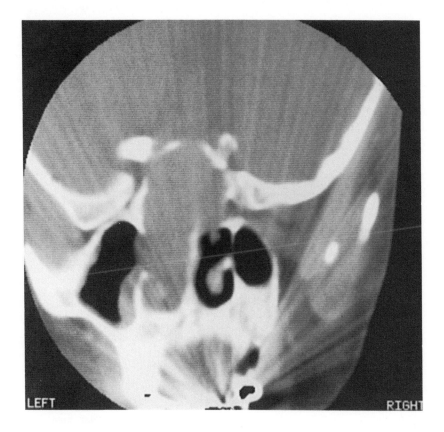

3 Cardiovascular and Lymphatic Systems

The heart

METHODS OF INVESTIGATION

Imaging investigations play a significant role in diagnostic cardiology, and include the following methods.

Plain radiographs
Films of the chest show the size, shape, and position of the heart and, equally importantly, the state of the lungs and pulmonary vessels. Cardiac calcifications may be visible, but individual chamber sizes are difficult to assess reliably.

Ultrasound.
Not only can morphology and movement of the heart be demonstrated, but patterns of blood flow and especially shunts and valvular regurgitation may be measured. It is particularly useful in small children.

Nuclear medicine
Computer aided scanning is playing an increasing role in the detection of recent and old myocardial infarcts, or ischaemia, and in the non-invasive measurement of intracardiac shunts, segmental wall movement, and ejection fractions.

Angiocardiography
This remains the 'gold standard' in the assessment of many diseases, but the continuing development of accurate non-invasive methods is reducing its use.

Coronary angiography
This is the only current method of providing detailed anatomical information on the coronary arteries, and remains an essential investigation if surgery is contemplated.

LESIONS OF THE HEART

HEART FAILURE
This is one of the most common of clinical problems and a plain chest radiograph is an essential part of the initial work-up. While the appearances of pulmonary oedema have already been described in the 'Chest' section (Chapter 2) reiteration with emphasis on chest radiography in heart failure is warranted.

1. The size of the heart shadow is easily seen on postero-anterior views, which, for proper comparison, should be made with the patient erect and with good inspiratory effort (Figure 3.1). The ratio between cardiac and thoracic diameters should be less than 70% in children and 50% in adults (Figure 3.2). It should be noted that, although cardiac enlargement is usual in heart failure due to ventricular disease, it may not occur in some cases of cardiogenic

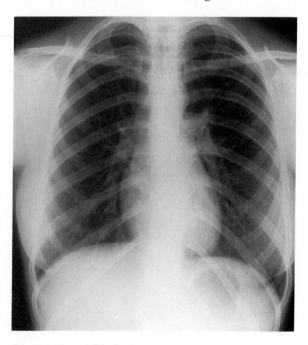

Fig. 3.1 Normal PA chest.

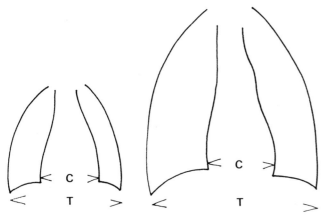

Fig. 3.2 Cardio-thoracic ratio. In adults, normally C/T < 0.5, in infants, normally C/T < 0.7 (depending on age)

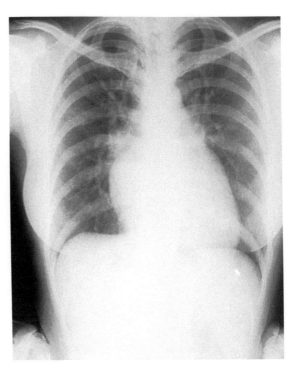

Fig. 3.3 Enlarged upper lobe veins in raised pulmonary venous pressure.

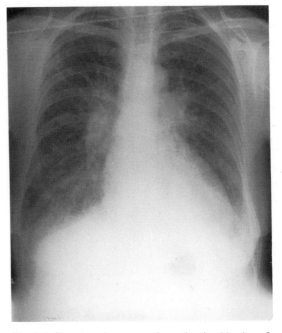

Fig. 3.4 Chronic pulmonary oedema showing blurring of hilar outlines.

pulmonary oedema, e.g. occasionally in mitral valve disease, or in constrictive pericarditis.

2. Pulmonary vessels, arteries, and veins normally comprise almost all the markings in the lungs. The upper lobe vessels are normally small compared with those of the lower lobes (an effect of gravity). The vessels should be noted to taper and branch as they pass out into the lungfields and be visible to about 2 cm from the chest wall.

The normal calibre of lung vessels should be appreciated, since detection of pulmonary oligaemia (as in pulmonary atresia, page 70) or plethora (as in left to right shunts e.g. atrial septal defect) is mandatory to arrive at a correct diagnosis. Furthermore, enlargement of upper lobe vessels relative to lower lobe vessels (Figure 3.3) (with the patient erect) is strong evidence of elevated pulmonary venous pressure, or, less commonly, grossly increased pulmonary artery blood flow. Destruction or obstruction of lower lobe vessels (basal emphysema or emboli) gives the same appearance.

3. Pulmonary oedema as related to heart disease takes two principal forms:

(a) Chronic pulmonary oedema with increased upper lobe vessel diameter, Kerley B lines (indicating interlobular septal lymph engorgement), hilar blurring and enlargement, and sometimes pleural effusions (Figure 3.4).

(b) Acute pulmonary oedema may arise *de novo* or be superimposed on chronic oedema. The radiological appearances include perihilar bat's wing opacities and occasionally pleural effusions (Figure 3.5). There will usually be Kerley B lines only with pre-existing chronic oedema. It should be noted that heart failure is only one of many causes of acute pulmonary oedema (see Chapter 2).

Heart failure, usually left ventricular failure, is thus classically characterized by a large heart, enlarged upper lobe vessels and the signs, as appropriate, of acute or chronic pulmonary oedema.

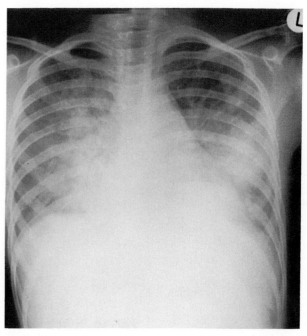

Fig. 3.5 Acute pulmonary oedema with 'bat's wing' appearance.

CONGENITAL ANOMALIES

The range of congenital cardiac anomalies is vast, ranging from atrial septal defects through other left-to-right shunts to valvular and chamber aplasias and malrotations. Only the most common of the major groups will be described.

Non-cyanotic congenital heart disease

Typically, this is due to an atrial septal defect, ventricular septal defect, or patent ductus arteriosus, which often present as asymptomatic heart murmurs.

Radiological appearances

1. Plain radiograph: this may show a normal or enlarged heart size with prominence of the main pulmonary artery (Figure 3.6). The lungfields will show normal vascularity, or if the shunt is large, plethora, differentiating the lesion from pulmonary valve stenosis (page 70).

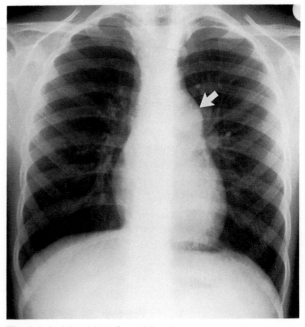

Fig. 3.6 Atrial septal defect with pulmonary artery prominence (→).

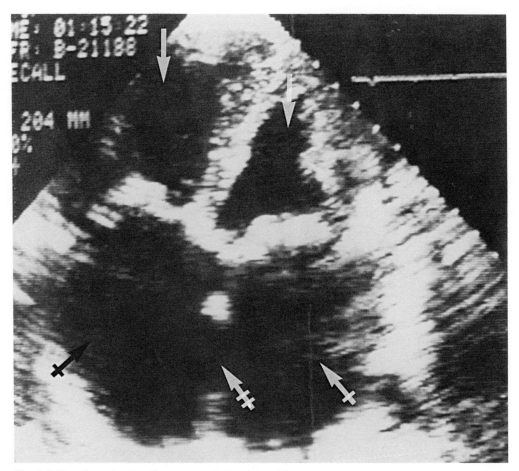

Fig. 3.7 Two-dimensional cardiac ultrasound, showing atrial septal defect. Ventricles (→), atria (↔), septal defect (⇸).

2. Ultrasound: differential contraction of the right and left ventricles and higher flow rates in the right heart may be demonstrated. A septal defect may be visualized directly (Figure 3.7).

3. Nuclear medicine: this may be useful to quantitate shunts non-invasively by measuring relative flow and recirculation in the lungs (Figure 3.8). Radionuclide angiography may also indicate the anatomical state in complicated defects.

4. Cardiac catheterization: this allows the measurement of pressures, oximetry, dye studies, and angiocardiography and remains the 'gold standard' for investigation but, as non-invasive tests become more versatile and accurate, tends to be used more selectively.

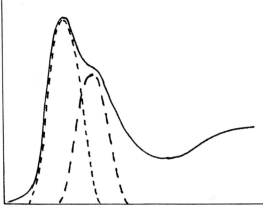

Fig. 3.8 Nuclear medicine shunt assessment. Activity/time from right lung. Detected lung activity after intravenous injection (—). Computed first pass through lung (----). Computed recirculation through lung (– – –). Shunt ratio = 1.8 : 1.

Cyanotic congenital heart disease

This typically includes complex defects, with chamber, valve, or vessel hypoplasia or malrotation. The complexity often requires multiple tests for elucidation, especially if surgery is contemplated.

The most common cyanotic congenital defect is the pulmonary dysplasia group typified by Fallot's tetralogy (Figure 3.9).

Radiological appearances

1. Plain chest radiographs: these characteristically show an enlarged heart with right ventricular prominence, absent or small pulmonary artery segment, and oligaemic lung fields. A right-sided aortic arch may also be present. Absence of the spleen indicates a complex lesion.

2. Ultrasound shows the thickened right ventricle and may show the pulmonary outflow tract hypoplasia and abnormal valves.

3. Cardiac catheterization and angiocardiography are required for detailed analysis prior to surgery.

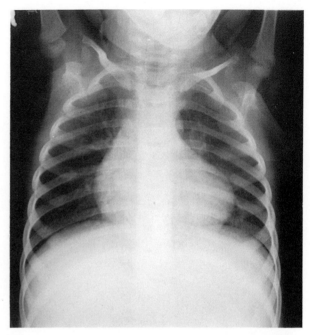

Fig. 3.9 Fallot's tetralogy.

Pulmonary stenosis

This may be due to hypoplasia with right to left shunting, but may also be due to congenital stenosis of the pulmonary valve (Figure 3.10).

Radiological appearances

1. Plain radiographs: a normal or large heart, with a prominent pulmonary artery segment (due to post-stenotic dilatation) and normal or oligaemic lungfields.

2. Ultrasound shows a thickened right ventricular wall and failure of opening of the domed pulmonary valve.

3. Cardiac catheterization shows raised right ventricular pressures, with a large drop across the stenotic valve, and on angiography the domed narrow valve is clearly shown.

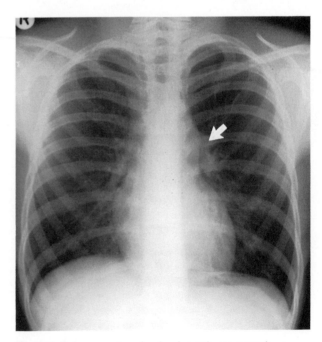

Fig. 3.10 Pulmonary stenosis, showing pulmonary trunk prominence (→), and lung oligaemia.

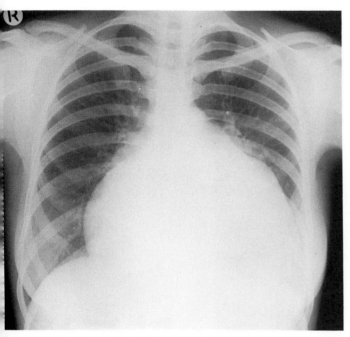

Fig. 3.11 Cardiac enlargement in myocarditis.

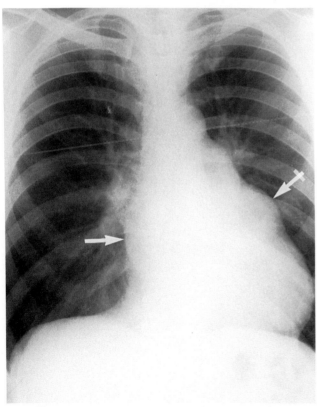

Fig. 3.12 Mitral valve disease, showing enlarged left atrium; right border (→) and atrial appendage (↔).

TRAUMA

Injury to the heart is rare except in road traffic accidents and penetrating wounds. Imaging is generally not useful except in the detection of associated haemopericardium, when ultrasound in particular is of great value.

INFLAMMATORY

Myocarditis

This may be viral or degenerative (e.g. alcoholic myocarditis) or occasionally auto-immune.

Radiological appearances
1. Plain radiographs show a large heart and in many cases evidence of heart failure of variable severity (Figure 3.11)
2. Fluoroscopy shows poor contractility.
3. Ultrasound shows enlarged chambers and poor contractility.
4. Nuclear medicine shows large chambers and reduced ejection fraction (normal is greater than 55%).

Endocarditis

This is usually associated with either rheumatic fever (with myocarditis) or bacterial infections. The valves in particular are often involved, with stenosis and/or incompetence following rheumatic fever and in bacterial endocarditis eventual destruction and incompetence. The most commonly affected valves are the mitral and aortic.

Mitral valve disease

Radiological appearances
1. Plain radiographs: The heart size varies from normal to huge, the chamber enlargement being primarily left atrial with prominence of the right heart border and atrial appendage. Raised pulmonary venous pressure produces relatively enlarged upper lobe vessels (Figure 3.12). Evidence of pulmonary oedema may vary from nil, through Kerley's lines, to full-blown acute oedema. Back pressure to the right heart will produce enlargement of the pulmonary

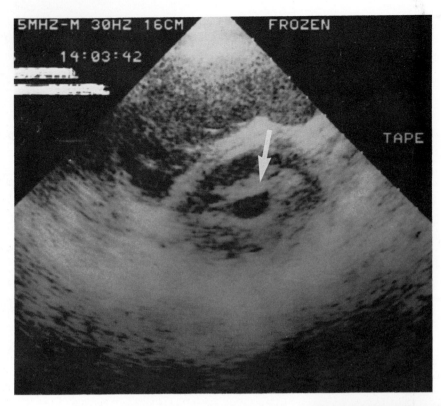

A

Fig. 3.13 (A) Two-dimensional ultrasound in mitral stenosis
showing thickened valve with narrow orifice.
(B) M-mode ultrasound in mitral valve stenosis.

artery trunk and right ventricle. Advanced cases
may show valve calcification.

2. Ultrasound shows the stiffened and
stenosed mitral valve clearly and is often the
only additional test needed (Figure 3.13).

3. Cardiac catheterization was normally
performed pre-operatively to assess the degree of
stenosis, but is now to a considerable extent
replaced by ultrasound.

Aortic valve disease
This may be congenital or acquired as a result
of either degeneration or inflammatory disease as
above.

Radiological appearances
1. *Plain radiographs* show cardiac enlargement,
typically affecting principally the left ventricle
which shows as extension of the heart shadow to
the left at the apex. Valve calcification may be

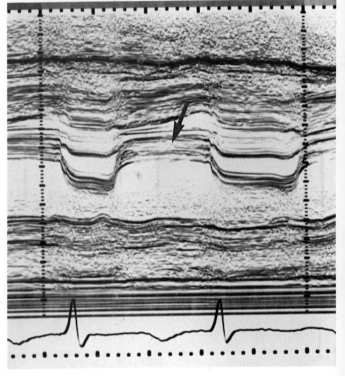

B

seen. If cardiac failure supervenes, the radiographic features (page 66) will appear.

2. Ultrasound and cardiac catheterization are applicable and valuable as in mitral valve disease.

Acute pericarditis

This condition is usually characterized by the presence of a pericardial effusion.

RADIOLOGICAL APPEARANCES

1. Plain radiographs will show an enlarged heart shadow (often occurring acutely) (Figure 3.14). The appearance is essentially indistinguishable from myocarditis or left ventricular failure. The signs of pulmonary oedema may be seen. (Fluoroscopy will demonstrate little cardiac movement.)

2. Ultrasound is by far the most useful test and has effectively replaced all other tests for pericardial effusion by demonstrating the fluid in the pericardial sac (Figure 3.15).

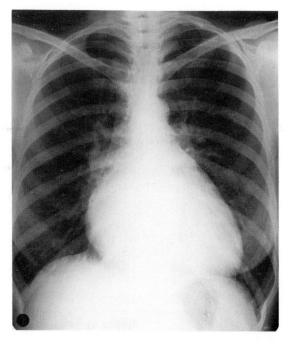

Fig. 3.14 Enlarged cardiac outline in pericardial effusion.

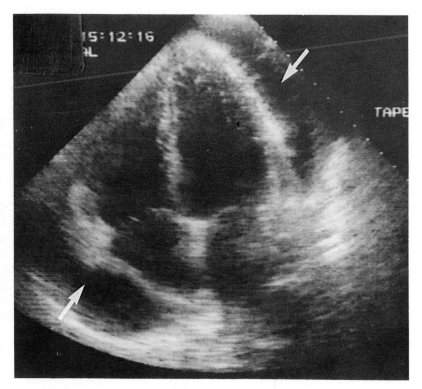

Fig. 3.15 Two-dimensional ultrasound in pericardial effusion.

Chronic pericarditis

This may present with fibrosis and constriction, with or without heart failure.

Radiological appearances

1. Plain radiographs will show a heart shadow of (usually) normal size. Extensive pericardial calcification is virtually pathognomonic but may not be present (Figure 3.16). Heart failure may also be present in some cases, depending on the predominance of chamber embarrassment.

2. Ultrasound shows the thickened pericardium and poor contraction.

ISCHAEMIA

Cardiac ischaemia and its sequelae are amongst the most common of severe ailments. The diagnosis is principally by clinical history, ECG with or without stress testing, and enzyme estimations. In a proportion of cases further tests are needed to clarify the fairly extensive differential diagnosis, and in all cases in which coronary artery by-pass grafting (CABG) is contemplated a thorough work-up is needed.

Radiological appearances

1. Plain radiographs: these are usually non-contributory but may show coronary artery calcification, cardiomegaly and evidence of pulmonary oedema.

2. Coronary artery angiography (CAA) is the anatomical test *par excellence* for demonstrating the state of these vessels and is used both diagnostically and in pre-CABG work-up (Figure 3.17).

3. Ultrasound: the contractility of the left and right ventricles can be shown, but it may be difficult to perform in obese or emphysematous subjects.

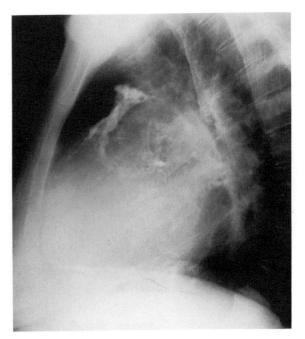

Fig. 3.16 Pericardial calcification.

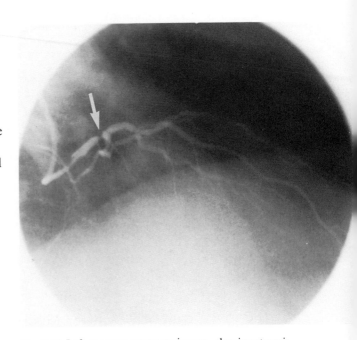

Fig. 3.17 Left coronary artery angiogram, showing stenosis.

4. Nuclear medicine. A variety of tests are available:

   (a) Regional myocardial perfusion by thallium chloride showing myocardial infarcts.

   (b) Uptake of Tc-99m pyrophosphate in recently infarcted tissue (Figure 3.18).

   (c) Blood pool scanning using Tc-99m labelled red cells, showing segmental contractility of the myocardium and accurate and reproducible measurement of the ejection fraction. An ejection fraction (EF) of less than 15% contraindicates further investigation.

See Diagnostic decision tree 2 (page 301), which relates to coronary insufficiency.

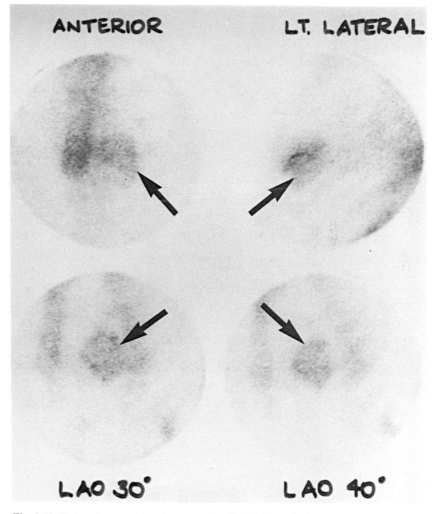

Fig. 3.18 Technetium pyrophosphate scan showing high uptake in recent myocardial infarct ($\rightarrow$). There is also uptake in bone.

Myocardial infarcts

These are generally easily diagnosed on clinical, ECG, or enzyme grounds, but on occasion, if admission is delayed or a left bundle branch block is present, further tests may be required.

The most appropriate, noted above, are nuclear medicine using infarct-avid Tc-99m pyrophosphate, and perhaps nuclear medicine blood pool studies showing myocardial regional dyskinesia (Figure 3.19).

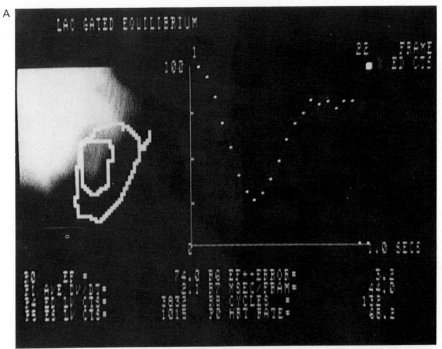

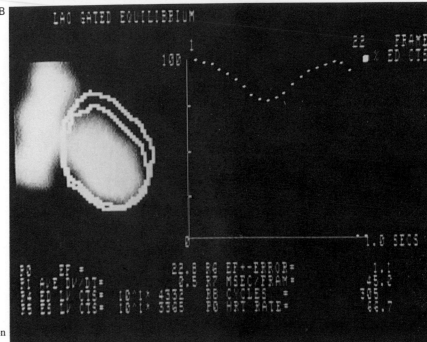

Fig. 3.19 Gated blood pool studies for ventricular function. (A) Normal left ventricular contraction, with 74% ejection fraction. (B) Left ventricular contraction after infarct. Ejection fraction 22%.

The aorta and peripheral vessels

A useful set of general rules governing the size of vessels is that the diameter of any vessel depends on:

1. The flow through the vessel (e.g. an enlarged pulmonary artery with atrial septal defect and right-to-left shunt; or a small renal artery in chronic pyelonephritis with a small hypofunctioning kidney).

2. The static (lateral) pressure in the vessel (e.g. post-stenotic dilatation due to turbulence).

3. The state of the vessel wall (e.g. an aneurysm associated with degeneration or injury; or stenosis due to atheromatous plaques).

The factors may operate singly or in any combination, e.g. in atrial septal defect both flow and pressure may be high in the pulmonary artery.

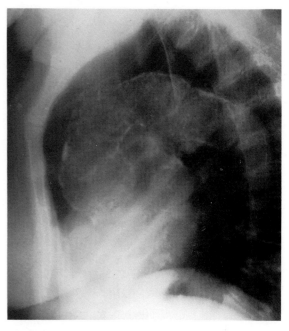

Fig. 3.20 Calcification in syphilitic aortic aneurysm.

METHODS OF INVESTIGATION

Plain radiographs
These are of considerable value in those circumstances in which the vessel is visible, e.g. the aortic arch outlined against lung and often with calcification in the wall (Figure 3.20). Enlargement, particularly when increasing, spells aneurysm. Elsewhere, vessels show against soft tissue only when the wall is calcified — a frequent appearance in degenerative disease of abdominal, pelvic and peripheral arteries.

Angiography
This examination with selective vessel catheterization as necessary demonstrates the vessel lumen in great detail. The low but significant risks of catheterization and large contrast injections are being reduced by the advent of digital subtraction angiography, which permits demonstration of the larger vessels by intravenous bolus injections or, alternatively, the use of smaller catheters and contrast volumes in arterial injections.

Ultrasound
This is especially useful in assessing the abdominal aorta non-invasively and, to a lesser extent, the other peripheral vessels. High resolution ultrasound with Doppler analysis of flow is becoming most helpful in the recognition of carotid artery stenosis.

Computerized tomography
This shows aneurysms of large vessels well but, as its demonstration of flow is very limited, it is of less value in showing lesions in smaller vessels.

Magnetic resonance imaging
This has great promise, especially if the flow is measurable.

Nuclear medicine
Gross information on vessel patency and relative

blood flow is provided, particularly in paired vessels, but the resolution is still inadequate for detailed anatomical studies.

Interventional techniques
These involve percutaneous catheter dilatation of stenosed vessels and occlusion of bleeding vessels or the feeders of arterio-venous malformations by artificial embolisation via a catheter (see Chapter 11).

LESIONS OF THE AORTA

Basically all vascular problems requiring investigation are either congenital (developmental) abnormalities, dilatations (aneurysms), abnormal communications (arterio-venous malformations or fistulae), stenoses (usually atheromatous), or occlusions (commonly thrombotic or embolic). The investigations required vary considerably depending on the provisional diagnosis and location of the lesion.

CONGENITAL LESIONS
These are principally developmental anomalies of the aortic arch, occasionally with a double or partially double arch producing a vascular ring which may cause oesophageal narrowing.

Coarctation of the aorta
The severity of the stenosis determines the signs and symptoms and whether treatment is necessary.

Radiological appearances
1. Plain radiographs will show the location of the aortic arch and may display the narrowing due to coarctation and its post-stenotic dilatation. Large intercostal anastomoses may produce rib notching (Figure 3.21).
2. Barium swallow demonstrates oesophageal narrowing by a vascular ring or deviation by post-coarctation dilatation.
3. Angiography shows the lesion definitively (Figure 3.22).

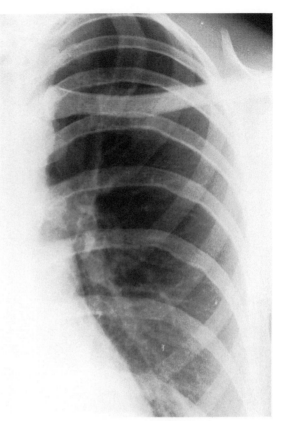

Fig. 3.21 Rib notching in coarctation of the aorta.

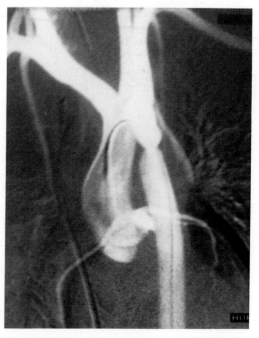

Fig. 3.22 Digital subtraction aortogram of coarctation of aorta.

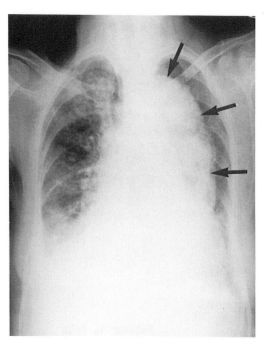

Fig. 3.23 PA chest showing aortic aneurysm.

ANEURYSMS

These are usually degenerative and fusiform in nature, although traumatic (usually road traffic accidents) and syphilitic aneurysms do occur. Any part of the aorta may be affected although syphilitic lesions have a predeliction for the ascending aorta, and degenerative lesions for the abdominal aorta, usually below the origin of the renal arteries.

Radiological appearances
  1. Plain radiographs: dilatation of the the thoracic aorta is clearly shown (Figure 3.23).
  2. Ultrasound is the primary investigation in abdominal aneurysms, showing the size, shape and position of the aneurysm and allowing simple regular follow-up (Figure 3.24). An aneurysm greater than 4 cm in diameter or increasing in size requires surgery unless there are strong contraindications.

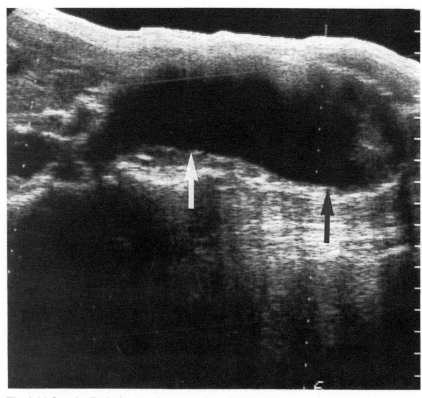

Fig. 3.24 Longitudinal ultrasound examination of abdominal aortic aneurysm (→).

3. Computerized tomography is very useful in all aortic aneurysms, especially to differentiate them from other causes of abdominal or mediastinal masses (Figure 3.25). Contrast infusion will show the lumen and thus the presence of any mural clots or dissections.

4. Angiography, although seldom used now, may be required in complex problems, especially if there is evidence of occlusion of branch vessels or if surgery is contemplated. The availability of digital subtraction angiography will lead to much wider use of this accurate and low-risk procedure.

Dissecting aneurysms

These are a cause of an acute chest or abdominal emergency, and are investigated in a similar manner to other aneurysms, although CT and angiography tend to be used early. A double lumen appearance is characteristic and spread of the dissection may occlude branch vessels such as the coronary and renal arteries.

LESIONS OF THE PERIPHERAL ARTERIES

The major branches of the aorta occasionally show aneurysm formation (particularly in renal and iliac arteries) and are investigated as for the aorta, but with the emphasis on angiography. The more common problem is stenosis or occlusion with distal ischaemia. The most commonly affected vessels are the carotids, usually at the origin of the internal carotids (see Chapter 7), and the ilio-femoral vessels supplying the lower limb.

ISCHAEMIA

Carotid ischaemia gives rise to strokes or transient ischaemic attacks, and leg ischaemia to claudication and, in severe cases, to ulcers or gangrene.

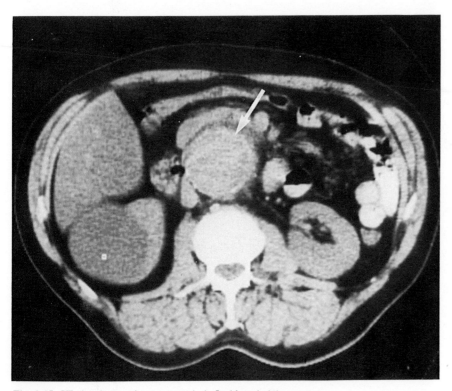

Fig. 3.25 CT showing aortic aneurysm (→). Incidental right renal cyst.

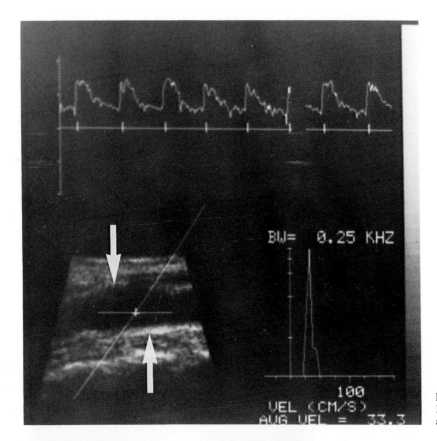

Fig. 3.26 Ultrasound and Doppler graph of normal carotid artery.

Radiological appearances

1. Ultrasound: the use of high resolution systems with Doppler flow analysis is particularly useful in the investigation of the carotids (Figure 3.26). Other arteries are less amenable to ultrasound due largely to their relatively greater depth from the skin.

2. Angiography: when performed with or without digital subtraction, this is the mainstay of investigation (Figure 3.27). Techniques of percutaneous catheterization are such that virtually any artery can be selected for localized study as required. Aneurysms, stenoses, or occlusions are clearly shown together with any collaterals which may have formed. Fistulae or arterio-venous malformations are also clearly shown.

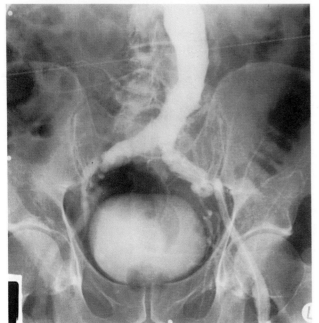

Fig. 3.27 Arteriogram of lower aorta and pelvic vessels showing iliac artery stenoses.

SMALL VESSEL DISEASE

This is usually associated with Buerger's disease, sub-acute lupus erythematosus, Raynaud's or similar diseases and may be studied by angiography, using selective approaches and magnification radiography. Such study, however, is rarely necessary for diagnostic or therapeutic purposes.

ARTERIO-VENOUS FISTULAE

These are usually traumatic or mycotic in origin. The presence of a thrill and bruit is usually diagnostic, but angiography is required to define the lesion and its feeding arteries and draining veins prior to surgery. Pulmonary arteries suffer from similar disease processes.

LESIONS OF VEINS

The major lesions involving veins are aneurysm or incompetence (varicose veins), phlebitis, thrombosis, or occlusion by extrinsic pressure.

VARICOSE VEINS

These principally affect the leg. Imaging is generally not required in the diagnosis or treatment, but in some cases of recurrent varicosities a search for incompetent perforating veins by venography may be profitable. Venography is performed by injection of contrast medium into a vein on the dorsum of the foot, while occluding the superficial veins at the ankle by a tight bandage or tourniquet. The deep veins are thus filled and any passage of the contrast medium to the superficial veins indicates and localizes the incompetent perforating veins.

DEEP VEIN THROMBOSIS

This is common, especially post-operatively and is the prime cause of pulmonary embolism.

Radiological appearances

1. Venography: non-filling of deep veins or clots within the lumen are shown (Figure 3.28). It is probably the most accurate single test.

2. Nuclear medicine: blood pool scanning is reasonably sensitive for deep vein thrombosis, showing as poor or absent filling of the deep veins. It is useful as a non-invasive technique when, due to infection or oedema, there is difficulty in cannulating a foot vein to perform venography.

3. Ultrasound: when used with Doppler this will indicate venous obstruction, particularly in the popliteal and femoral veins.

VENOUS OBSTRUCTION

This usually affects the iliac veins, inferior vena cava, superior vena cava, renal, or subclavian veins following trauma, radiation therapy, or extrinsic pressure (often due to neoplastic masses). Occasionally it occurs spontaneously.

Radiological appearances

1. Venography: injection of contrast medium into the appropriate limb or central veins will show the obstruction and the passage of blood and contrast through collaterals.

2. Nuclear medicine venography: this will give the same information, with less spatial resolution, using a radionuclide rather than a contrast injection.

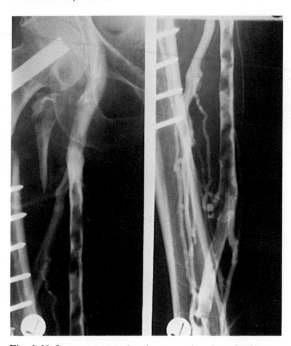

Fig. 3.28 Leg venogram showing extensive thrombosis.

The spleen

METHODS OF INVESTIGATION

Plain radiographs
Plain abdominal radiographs provide a useful
primary investigation and often (but not always)
show the size and shape of the spleen. With
enlargement of the spleen there is displacement
of the stomach air bubble and sometimes of the
left kidney.

Angiography
Splenic arteriography is rarely used for
investigation of the spleen itself except in cases
of trauma, but usually as part of a study of the
portal system as in portal hypertension.

Ultrasound
The spleen is usually well seen and its size may
be estimated. Splenic ruptures may be well
shown, especially if there is a perisplenic
haematoma present.

Radionuclide scan
Being a reticulo-endothelial structure, the spleen
concentrates foreign materials, such as labelled
colloids (see liver scanning, page 128) and
labelled damaged red cells. A radionuclide scan
is therefore particularly useful as a non-invasive
method of showing the size, shape, position and
function of this organ (Figure 3.29).

STATIC LIVER STUDY

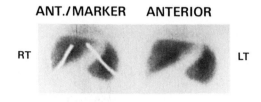

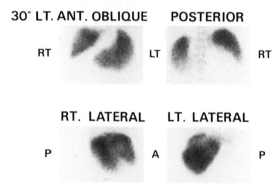

DOSE: 2mCi of ^{99m}TC S/C, given I.V.

Fig. 3.29 Radionuclide scan of liver and spleen, using
technetium-99m labelled sulphur colloid.

Computerized tomography
This shows the spleen and perisplenic collections well and, more importantly, shows any lymphomatous lesions in the retroperitoneal tissues (Figure 3.30).

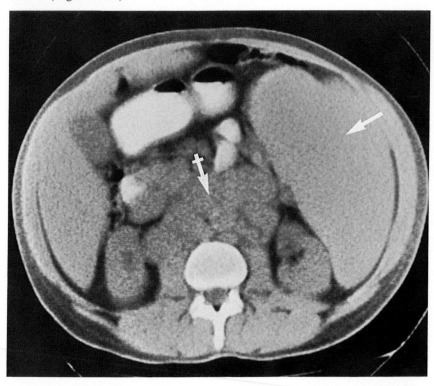

Fig. 3.30 Abdominal CT in case of lymphoma, showing enlarged spleen (→) and para-aortic lymph nodes (↔).

LESIONS OF THE SPLEEN

CONGENITAL
Asplenia is rare except in association with complex heart lesions. Polysplenia is also rare, but of importance in hypersplenism or following splenic injury. Both of these conditions are best seen by radionuclide scanning, although CT may be helpful.

TRAUMA
Splenic rupture is common, especially in children, and may lead to early or late torrential haemorrhage. Previously, orthodox treatment was by splenectomy but this is now done less commonly since healing can be shown on serial imaging studies in a high proportion of cases.

Radiological appearances
All the methods of investigation described previously are useful in trauma, but the most useful are the following:
1. Plain radiographs: signs of splenic injury may include elevation of the left hemidiaphragm, fracture of left lower rib(s), displacement of the stomach bubble to the right, obliteration of the left psoas shadow, and enlargement of the splenic outline (see Figure 5.8).
2. Radionuclide scan: multiple views will almost always show the tear in the spleen as well as any displacement of the organ due to a haematoma. Serial studies over a period may show healing.
3. Ultrasound: this may show a splenic and/or perisplenic haematoma.
4. Computerized tomography: although less commonly used, this is a good method of displaying perisplenic collections.

INFLAMMATORY

The spleen may be directly involved by infection in septicaemia, when it is large and soft. Malaria, typhoid fever, brucellosis, and tuberculosis may also involve the spleen, the latter occasionally producing calcified tubercles visible on plain radiographs.

SPLENOMEGALY

This is one of the common reasons for imaging investigations of the spleen. Splenomegaly has multiple causes.

Hypersplenism

Primary or secondary. All tests show splenic enlargement but radionuclide scanning will also demonstrate excessive labelled colloid or labelled red cell uptake, indicating the excess trapping (Figure 3.31). The degree of trapping and red cell destruction may also be measured by radionuclide labelled red cell techniques.

Infiltration

Amyloid disease and sarcoidosis are the common infiltrating conditions. There are no specific imaging signs, although discrete deposits may show as defects on radionuclide scanning.

Lipid storage diseases

All tests show splenomegaly with reduced uptake by the spleen in radionuclide scans.

Lymphoma

Splenomegaly is usually present and easily seen on all tests. The nature of the splenic enlargement is usually not determinable by imaging, although the presence of enlarged lymph nodes, either clinically or on computerized tomography, provides a valuable clue. Chest manifestations of lymphoma are relatively common (see Chapter 2).

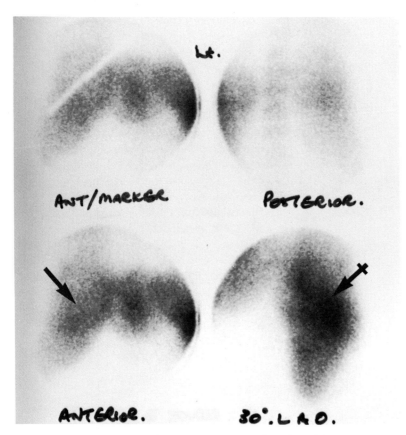

Fig. 3.31 Radionuclide scan of enlarged and hyperactive spleen: Liver (→), Spleen (↔).

Lymphatics and lymph nodes

METHODS OF INVESTIGATION

Plain radiographs
Enlarged mediastinal and hilar lymph nodes are visible on a chest x-ray but, unless calcified, nodes are rarely visible elsewhere in the body.

Lymphography
Opaque material, usually Lipiodol Ultrafluide®, is injected over several hours into a peripheral lymphatic which has been cannulated. This technique shows both the lymphatics in the limb injected and the nodes in the draining chain which for the leg includes the pelvic and para-aortic nodes. Enlarged or infiltrated nodes may be seen.

Computerized tomography
This shows enlarged nodes, especially the hilar, mediastinal, retroperitoneal, and pelvic groups, and is the examination of choice in the diagnosis and staging of lymphomas.

Radionuclide scanning
Nuclear medicine lymphography may help in the examination of the internal mammary chain.

LESIONS OF THE LYMPHATICS

CONGENITAL
The only significant congenital lesion is Milroy's disease in which hypoplasia of lymphatics leads to oedema of the lower limbs. The paucity of lymphatic channels is well seen on lymphography.

INFLAMMATORY
Lymphoid enlargement may be due to inflammatory disease. It can be a potent cause of enlarged lung hilar nodes especially in children and must be differentiated from neoplastic involvement.

LYMPHOMAS
The lymphomas involve not only the lymph nodes but also the spleen, thymus, and other tissues.

Radiological appearances
1. Plain chest radiographs: hilar or mediastinal node enlargement or lung infiltration is shown.
2. Computerized tomography: scanning of the chest and abdomen may show enlargement of hilar, mediastinal or retroperitoneal nodes and spleen. This is the imaging investigation of choice for the detection and staging of lymphomas.
3. Lymphography: a characteristic lymph node pattern may be seen in Hodgkin's disease and non-specific abnormalities in other lymphomas (Figure 3.32).
   Metastatic deposits of tumour in lymph nodes are common in many neoplasms.

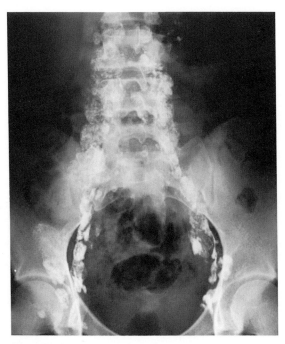

Fig. 3.32 Lymphogram showing enlarged foamy nodes in lymphoma.

Radiological appearances

1. Computerized tomography: node enlargement may be seen.

2. Ultrasound also shows enlarged nodes but less reliably.

3. Lymphography: there may be enlarged nodes with multiple filling defects, or with severe involvement there may be non-filling of the nodes (Figure 3.33).

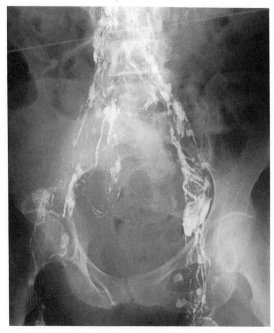

Fig. 3.33 Lymphogram with non-filling of pelvic nodes due to replacement by metastatic tumour.

Thymus

The thymus is normally large in infants, increases slightly in size in children, and becomes small in adult life.

METHODS OF INVESTIGATION

Plain radiographs
In infants the gland fills the anterior mediastinum and often appears as a mass with 'sail-like' margins (Figure 3.34). Recognition is necessary to prevent unnecessary treatment. The normal gland is rarely if ever seen in adults, but masses of thymic origin may mimic lymph node masses or aneurysms of the ascending aorta in the anterior mediastinum. (See pages 56, 57.)

Computerized tomography
This frequently shows the normal adult gland and demonstrates enlargements clearly.

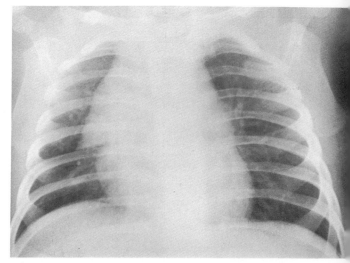

Fig. 3.34 Sail-shaped shadow of thymus in an infant.

LESIONS OF THE THYMUS

The only significant thymic lesions are tumours, which appear as masses in the anterior mediastinum and may be seen best on computerized tomography scans (Figure 3.35).

Fig. 3.35 Thoracic CT scan showing thymic mass in anterior mediastinum (→).

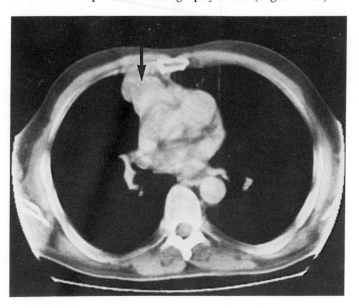

4 Alimentary Tract

Salivary glands

METHODS OF INVESTIGATION

Plain radiographs
Calculi in the glands or ducts are visible on plain films.

Sialography
Contrast medium injected into the ducts of the parotid and sub-maxillary glands will demonstrate the ducts within and outside the glands (Figure 4.1).

LESIONS OF SALIVARY GLANDS

SALIVARY CALCULI
Approximately 80% of calculi are visible on radiographs because they contain calcium carbonate (Figure 4.2).

SIALECTASIS
Dilatation of the ducts within the gland. It is usually the result of duct obstruction due to a calculus, with or without infection (Figure 4.3).

NEOPLASMS

Mixed salivary tumours
The gland is enlarged and the intra-glandular ducts are displaced.

Carcinoma
There is destruction of as well as displacement of ducts within the gland.

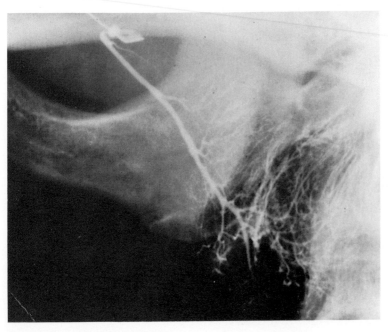

Fig. 4.1 Normal parotid sialogram.

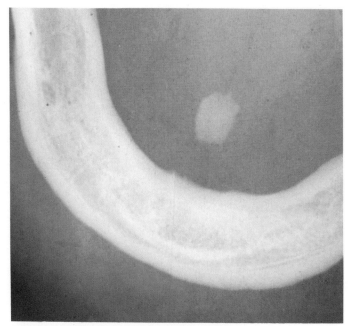

Fig. 4.2 Opaque calculus in submandibular gland duct.

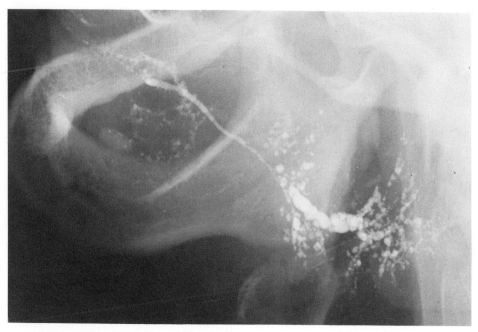

Fig. 4.3 Parotid sialectasis shown by sialography.

Pharynx

METHODS OF INVESTIGATION

Plain radiographs
Soft tissue lateral views show the pharynx well.

Tomography
This will often show the pharynx and any abnormality more clearly than will plain films.

Computerized tomography
CT is very useful for demonstrating soft tissue masses, and any associated bone involvement.

Contrast studies
1. Pharyngogram: contrast medium is instilled to outline the upper pharynx and any abnormality such as a tumour, which may be present.
2. Barium swallow: the lower pharynx is outlined by the barium sulphate suspension as the patient swallows.

LESIONS OF THE PHARYNX

DIVERTICULA
The most common is the Zenker's diverticulum which projects posteriorly between the transverse and oblique fibres of the inferior constrictor muscle and is readily seen with a barium swallow (Figure 4.4).

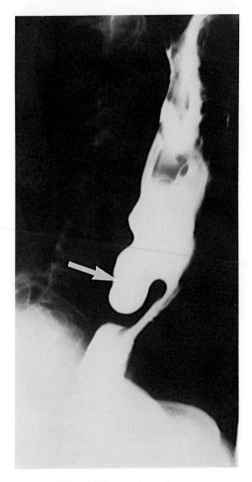

Fig. 4.4 Zenker's diverticulum of pharyngo-oesophageal junction (→). Barium swallow.

NEOPLASM

An irregular filling defect due to a neoplasm may be seen on the plain films or with contrast studies (Figure 4.5). Computerized tomography is useful to determine its extent.

RETROPHARYNGEAL ABSCESS

There is an increase in the thickness of the retropharyngeal soft tissues and forward displacement of the air-filled pharynx and the oesophagus (Figure 4.6).

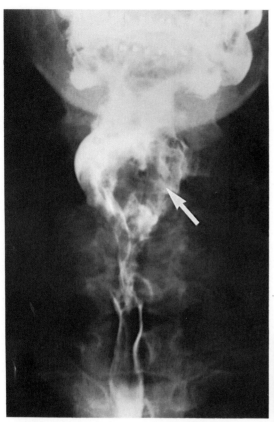

Fig. 4.5 Carcinoma of pharynx (→) shown on barium swallow.

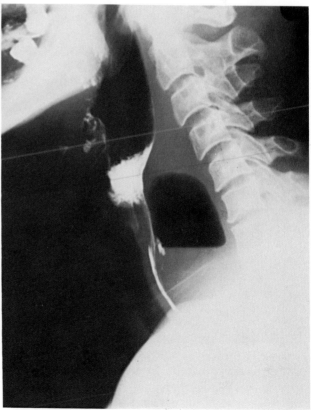

Fig. 4.6 Retropharyngeal abscess containing gas and liquid. Lateral view of barium swallow.

Oesophagus

METHODS OF INVESTIGATION

Plain radiographs
These may be used to demonstrate a foreign body in the oesophagus, or gas in the mediastinum following oesophageal perforation.

Contrast studies
The oesophagus is outlined by the patient swallowing a suspension of barium sulphate in water and this is the most common method of examination. It should *not* be used in cases where a foreign body is suspected or in cases where there may be a perforation of the oesophagus. A water-soluble contrast medium should be used under these circumstances because it is readily absorbed if it escapes into the lungs or through a perforation in the oesophageal wall.

An oily medium, lipiodol, or a water-soluble medium is used to examine the oesophagus in neonates for congenital abnormalities because of the possibility of the medium entering the trachea.

Computerized tomography
CT is reserved for the assessment of tumour extension.

NORMAL RADIOLOGICAL APPEARANCES

Under normal conditions the oesophagus can be seen only when filled with a contrast medium. It is then seen as a tube with parallel walls, with a smooth concave impression on the left border where the arch of the aorta presses on it and another, smaller, smooth indentation at the level at which the left main bronchus crosses the oesophagus. The distal end shows a short

segment of symmetrical smooth tapering where the oesophagus enters the hiatus in the diaphragm (Figure 4.7).

Peristaltic waves are not commonly seen with the patient erect but are visible when the patient is examined in the recumbent position, particularly if a thick barium cream is used.

The mucosal folds of the oesophagus appear as long, thin striations and are best seen at the lower end, but if the oesophagus is lined with gastric type mucous membrane (Barrett's mucosa) then the folds are coarse and irregular.

When barium is swallowed a phrenic ampulla may be seen as a localized dilated segment just above the diaphragm. This should not be confused with an hiatus hernia.

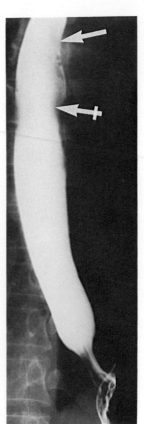

Fig. 4.7 AP view of normal oesophagus on barium swallow, showing aortic (→) and left bronchial (↔) impressions.

LESIONS OF THE OESOPHAGUS

CONGENITAL ABNORMALITIES OF THE OESOPHAGUS
These usually result from an abnormality in the separation of the trachea and oesophagus during development. This may result in the presence of a tracheo-oesophageal fistula, atresia, or a stricture of the oesophagus.

Fistula
Contrast can be seen to enter the trachea through the opening.

Atresia
Atresia shows as a smooth blunt termination of the oesophagus in the thorax (Figure 4.8); there is absence of gas in the stomach and bowel, and contrast may be seen to spill over the upper end of the oesophagus into the trachea.

Stricture
There is a smooth narrowing of the oesophagus.

DIVERTICULA
These may be single or multiple and can occur anywhere along the length of the oesophagus but are most common at the level of the lung hila. They appear as smooth, rounded, out-pouchings of the oesophagus in a barium swallow (Figure 4.9).

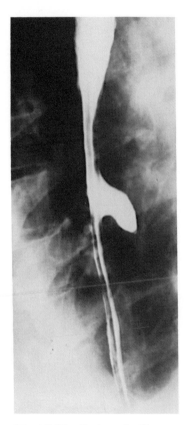

Fig. 4.9 Diverticulum of mid-oesophagus, on barium swallow.

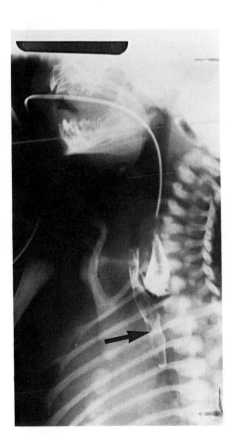

Fig. 4.8 Oesophageal atresia. Contrast administered by tube showing blind end of oesophagus, and spill into trachea (→).

STRICTURES

There are a number of causes of acquired oesophageal stricture.

Corrosive stricture

This results from swallowing corrosive substances and appears as a long, smooth, funnel-shaped narrowing of the oesophagus (Figure 4.10).

Reflux oesophagitis

This condition may be associated with peptic ulceration of the oesophagus and in these cases the ulcer crater may be seen in association with smooth narrowing of the oesophagus (Figure 4.11). If there is no peptic ulceration a smooth stricture of the oesophagus may occur. These strictures are usually associated with an hiatus hernia.

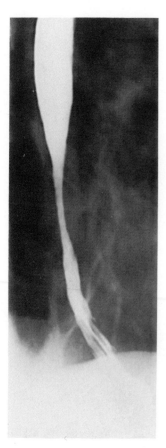

Fig. 4.10 Corrosive stricture of oesophagus, showing long smooth narrowing.

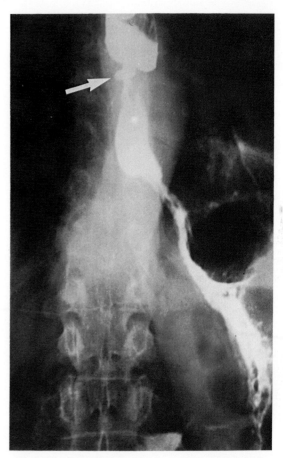

Fig. 4.11 Reflux oesophagitis with oesophageal ulcer (→) at barium meal.

Traumatic stricture
Usually long and smooth and may result from prolonged use of an indwelling gastric tube.

Malignant strictures
These are usually short and irregular (Figure 4.12), in distinction to all other strictures which are smooth. Occasionally, however, malignant strictures may be smooth, so that with all

strictures a biopsy should be taken by the endoscopist.

Vascular rings
These may cause narrowing due to extrinsic pressure.

VARICES
These usually occur at the lower end of the oesophagus and result from portal hypertension with dilatation of porto-systemic collaterals. They are seen as worm-like smooth filling defects in the contrast-filled oesophagus (Figure 4.13). Varices may also be demonstrated by filling the portal system with contrast medium during splenoportography (see Figure 5.7).

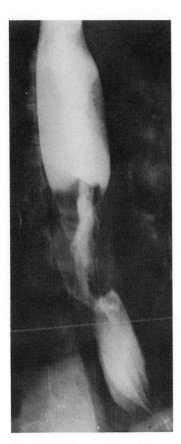

Fig. 4.12 Stricture of oesophagus due to carcinoma.

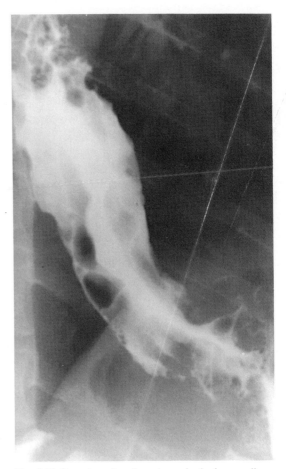

Fig. 4.13 Oesophageal varices shown by barium swallow.

NEOPLASMS

Benign tumours
These are usually leiomyomas or lipomas which appear as smooth filling defects in a contrast swallow.

Malignant tumours
Carcinoma is by far the most common malignant tumour. It has a predilection for three sites in the oesophagus:

1. Post-cricoid area. On the plain lateral view of the area the soft tissue space behind the cricoid, the width of which should not be more than the width of a cervical vertebra, is increased. In a contrast swallow examination the tumour appears as an irregular filling defect and is usually associated with delay in the passage of barium.

2. The level at which the left main bronchus crosses the oesophagus.

3. The lower one-third of the oesophagus. The tumours at the latter two sites usually appear as an area of marked irregularity of the oesophageal wall with narrowing of the lumen (see Figure 4.12). There is usually some dilatation of the oesophagus above the level of the lesion. However, particularly at the lower end of the oesophagus, the tumour may produce a smooth segment of narrowing with often marked dilatation of the oesophagus above this narrowing, and the appearances may closely simulate those of achalasia or benign stricture.

NEUROMUSCULAR ABNORMALITIES

Cork-screw oesophagus
With a barium swallow, the barium is segmented into multiple smooth sections. It may cause symptoms which mimic angina (Figure 4.14).

Cardiospasm (achalasia)
This results from failure of the cardiac sphincter to relax. The oesophagus becomes dilated, elongated and slow to empty. The distal end of the oesophagus is smooth and tapering (Figure 4.15), and there is usually an absence of gas in

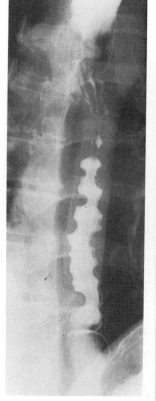

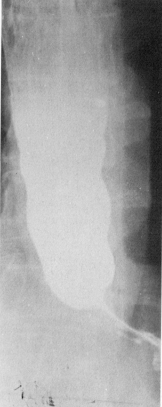

Fig. 4.14 Corkscrew oesophagus.

Fig. 4.15 Cardiospasm. The oesophagus is dilated, with stenosis at the lower end.

the fundus of the stomach. When the condition is advanced a plain film of the chest may show a smooth broadening of the mediastinal shadow and often a fluid level in the upper mediastinum due to air and fluid in the oesophagus.

In all cases biopsy from the wall of the oesophagus at the site of narrowing should be performed, since an intramural carcinoma may exactly simulate cardiospasm.

PERFORATION
This may result from instrumentation, a sharp foreign body, or prolonged vomiting. Gas may be seen in the mediastinum and contrast medium may escape through the perforation.

Water-soluble contrast medium must be used in the examination of cases of suspected perforation.

OESOPHAGEAL WEBS

These present as thin linear filling defects arising from the anterior wall of the upper oesophagus. They are visible in the lateral view of a contrast swallow (Figure 4.16). They may be associated with dysphagia and iron-deficiency anaemia.

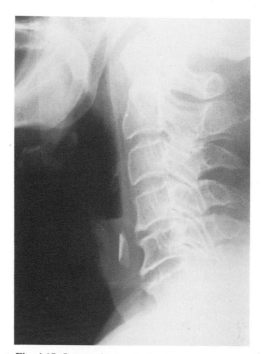

Fig. 4.17 Opaque foreign body (chop bone) in upper oesophagus.

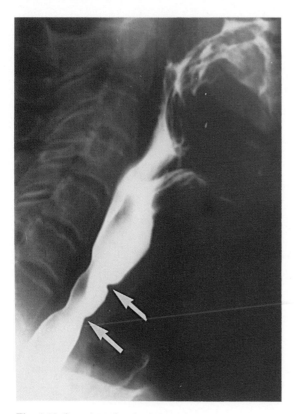

Fig. 4.16 Oesophageal webs (→). Lateral view of barium swallow.

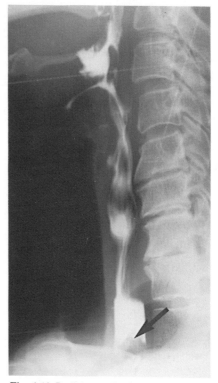

Fig. 4.18 Radiolucent foreign body in oesophagus outlined by contrast medium (→).

FOREIGN BODY

The majority of foreign bodies which become impacted do so in the cervical oesophagus. A plain lateral film of the neck may reveal the foreign body if it is radio-opaque (Figure 4.17). If nothing is seen on this film a water-soluble contrast (Gastrograffin®) swallow must be done. This may show the stream of contrast split by a radiolucent foreign body (Figure 4.18).

Stomach and duodenum

METHODS OF INVESTIGATION

Barium meal
The patient is given a suspension of barium sulphate in water to drink and the stomach and duodenum are examined.

Gas contrast barium meal
This method of examination is now most commonly used. After the patient has drunk a small quantity of barium suspension an effervescent tablet or drink is swallowed. The stomach and duodenum are thus distended with gas and the small quantity of barium is used simply to coat the walls of these structures.

Plain radiographs
These are occasionally used, particularly in infants. Absence of gas in the stomach in cases of oesophageal atresia, or a double fluid level due to gas and fluid in the fundus of the stomach and the duodenal cap may be shown when the baby is in the erect position, in cases of a congenital obstructive lesion of the duodenum.

NORMAL RADIOLOGICAL APPEARANCES

Examination of the contrast-containing stomach shows that the lesser curvature is smooth and sharply defined, whereas the greater curvature is often markedly irregular due to the folds of mucosa which project into the lumen but which may be obliterated when the stomach is distended with gas during the examination. The fundus is also smooth (Figure 4.19).

Peristaltic waves appear as smooth segments of narrowing in which the greater and lesser curvatures are symmetrically involved.

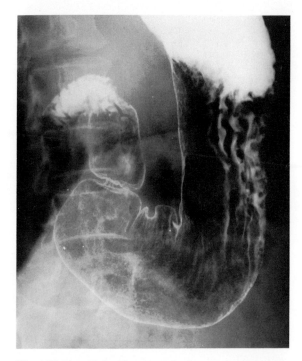

Fig. 4.19 Normal double contrast barium study of stomach.

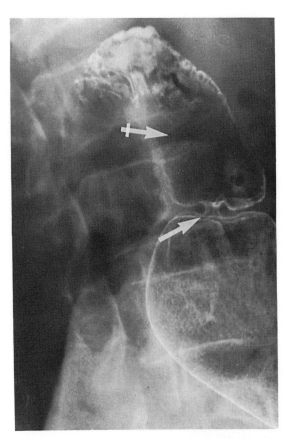

The pyloric canal is seen as a short thin line of contrast between the pyloric antrum and the first part of the duodenum. The first part of the duodenum when filled with barium is seen to be triangular and sitting symmetrically on the pyloric canal (Figure 4.20). It is called the duodenal cap because it resembles a tricorn hat.

The C-shaped curve of the duodenum surrounds the head of the pancreas and there is often a small out-pouching of the medial wall of the second part at the level of the ampulla of Vater.

The mucosa of the duodenum has many folds which disperse barium into a feather-like pattern (Figure 4.21).

Fig. 4.20 Normal pyloric canal (→) and duodenal cap (↔) on double contrast barium meal.

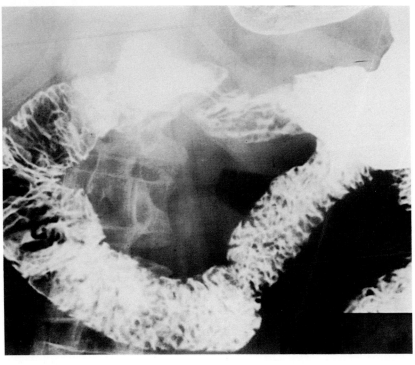

Fig. 4.21 Normal mucosal pattern of duodenal loop.

LESIONS OF THE STOMACH AND DUODENUM

CONGENITAL ABNORMALITIES

Congenital septa

These are seen most commonly in the second part of the duodenum, and may be complete or may have a small central orifice. They cause obstruction of the duodenum and a plain film with the patient erect may show the so-called 'double bubble' appearance which is due to air above fluid in the gastric fundus and the first part of the duodenum (Figure 4.22).

Diverticula

Congenital diverticula are rare in the stomach but when present are usually close to the oesophageal opening. They may be distinguished from ulcers by the fact that the gastric mucosal folds run into the diverticula but stop short of an ulcer crater. Diverticula of the duodenum are common and occur along the medial margin of this viscus (Figure 4.23).

Hypertrophic pyloric stenosis

The hypertrophic ring of muscle results in narrowing and elongation of the pyloric canal and indents both the pyloric antrum and the base of the duodenal cap to produce a shoulder deformity at each end of the pyloric canal (Figure 4.24).

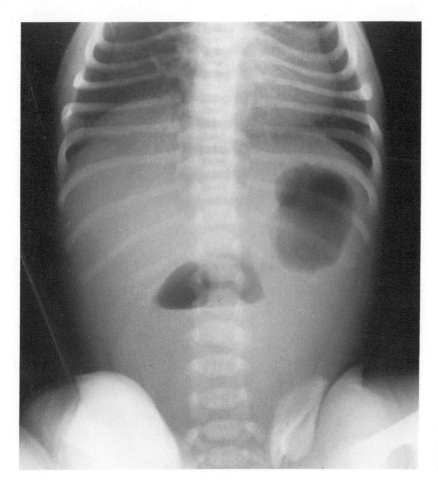

Fig. 4.22 'Double bubble' appearance in plain film of neonatal abdomen, due to duodenal atresia.

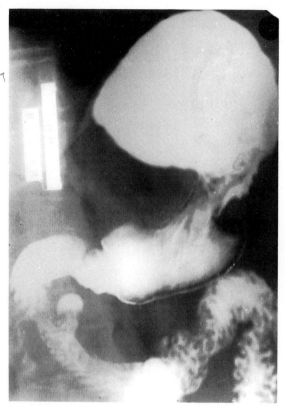

Fig. 4.23 Duodenal diverticulum.

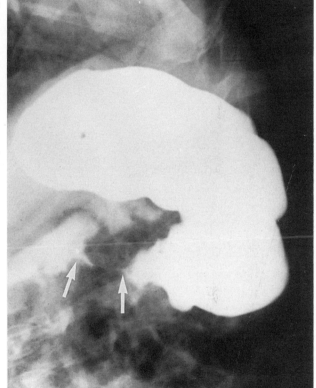

Fig. 4.24 Infantile pyloric
stenosis at barium meal. The
length of the pyloric canal is
shown ($\rightarrow$).

VOLVULUS

Volvulus of the stomach is most frequently seen
in patients with a large diaphragmatic hernia.
The stomach rotates so that the greater
curvature comes to lie uppermost and the
pyloric antrum and duodenal cap point
downwards. It also occurs if the left diaphragm
is markedly elevated, e.g. eventration.

GASTRIC ULCER

The most common site for peptic ulceration of
the stomach is on the anterior or posterior wall
of the stomach close to the lesser curvature.
Acute superficial ulceration is not a radiological
diagnosis because the ulcers are often too
shallow to be demonstrated.

Chronic ulcers penetrate the gastric wall and

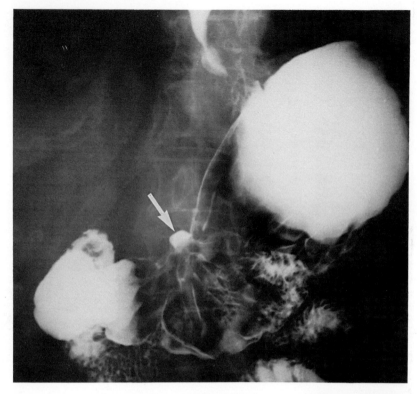

Fig. 4.25 Gastric ulcer in profile, at barium meal (→).

when seen in profile appear in a barium meal as
a rectangular collection of barium projecting
beyond the normal line of the margin of the
stomach (Figure 4.25). When seen *en face* they
appear as a central dot, surrounded by a zone
without mucosal folds due to oedema of the
mucosa.

With healing, the ulcer crater becomes smaller
and tends to be triangular; there may also be
extensive fibrosis, with resultant deformity of the
stomach. In the pyloric region this fibrosis may
lead to gastric outlet obstruction.

GASTRIC NEOPLASMS

Benign tumours
The common benign tumours are polyps arising
from mucosal glands, or leiomyomas from the
smooth muscle. They are smoothly rounded
(Figure 4.26). Occasionally an ulcer crater
develops on the surface of the tumour.

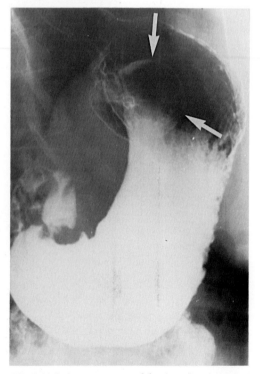

Fig. 4.26 Leiomyosarcoma of fundus of stomach (→).

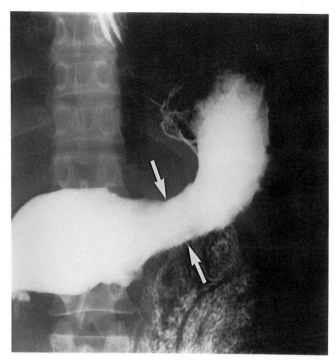

Fig. 4.27 Infiltrating carcinoma ('leather-bottle') stomach, (→) at barium meal.

Malignant tumours

Carcinoma is by far the most common malignant tumour although sarcomata do occur. There are three major presentations of carcinoma:

1. *Scirrhous or leather bottle*: Leather bottle stomach (linitus plastica) presents radiologically as a small, rigid, smoothly contracted stomach or segment of the stomach. It is aperistaltic (Figure 4.27).

2. *Fungating or encephaloid*: Fungating tumours show up in the barium meal as irregular filling defects with destruction of the overlying mucosa (Figure 4.28).

3. *Malignant ulcer*: the differentiation of benign and malignant ulcerative lesions depends on endoscopy and biopsy, and not on radiological appearances.

HIATUS HERNIA
See 'Diaphragmatic herniae', page 123.

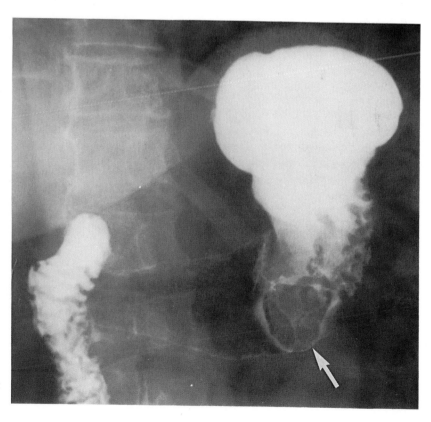

Fig. 4.28 Fungating carcinoma of stomach (→).

DUODENAL ULCER

The vast majority of ulcers occur in the first part of the duodenum (duodenal cap). Ulcers beyond the duodenal cap may occur following extensive burns or in the presence of a pancreatic islet cell tumour (Zollinger — Ellison Syndrome).

As with gastric ulcers, the ulcer crater may be demonstrated by a barium study (Figure 4.29). Quite commonly, however, the finding is only deformity of the duodenal cap. The cap is normally smoothly triangular but in the presence of ulceration and as the result of spasm and fibrosis it becomes irregular and often assumes a trefoil shape (Figure 4.30).

DUODENAL NEOPLASMS

Benign tumours

These are usually adenomatous polyps and are smooth and rounded.

Malignant tumours

Carcinoma rarely occurs in the first part of the duodenum. In the second part of the duodenum carcinoma may arise from the wall of the duodenum, from the ampulla of Vater, or from invasion by a carcinoma of the head of the pancreas. In each case there is a segment of irregular narrowing of the lumen and destruction of the mucosal pattern. A reversed 3 appearance on the medial wall of the second part of the duodenum results from a neoplasm of the head of the pancreas indenting the wall above and below the ampulla.

HAEMATEMESIS AND MELAENA

Haematemesis and melaena are symptoms often associated with oesophageal, gastric or duodenal pathology. A suggested imaging examination sequence for these symptoms is outlined in Diagnostic decision trees 3 and 4, pages 302 and 303.

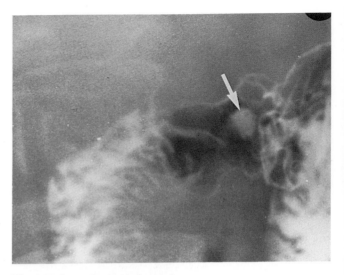

Fig. 4.29 Acute duodenal ulcer (→).

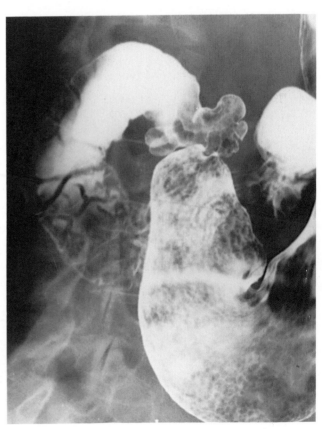

Fig. 4.30 Trefoil deformity of duodenal cap due to previous ulceration and scarring.

The small bowel

METHODS OF INVESTIGATION

Plain radiographs
When there is an ileus present *both erect and supine films of the abdomen must be made* and these show fluid levels and gas-distended loops. Plain films may also demonstrate a single gas-containing loop (sentinel loop) in an area of acute inflammatory change such as with pancreatitis. Plain films also enable a distinction to be made between obstructed small and large bowel.

Barium meal follow-through
After the contrast medium has left the stomach the barium-containing small bowel can be examined.

Small bowel enema
This examination greatly surpasses the follow-through technique. A tube is passed down to the duodeno-jejunal flexure and a dilute barium suspension instilled through the tube to fill the small bowel under fluoroscopic control.

Large bowel enema
The terminal ileum is often filled by reflux through the ileo-colic valve during a barium enema.

Arteriography
This is sometimes used to find a bleeding point in the bowel and artificial embolisation may be performed to arrest the bleeding.

Radionuclide scan
Technetium pertechnate is concentrated by gastric mucosa and may sometimes demonstrate a Meckel's diverticulum if it contains this type of mucosa.

NORMAL RADIOLOGICAL APPEARANCES

Plain radiographs
Normally the plain films do not show the small bowel or its contents apart perhaps from small quantities of gas.

Barium study
Barium in the duodenum has a feathery pattern. The valvulae conniventes are numerous in the upper part of the small bowel and become less numerous as the bowel is followed down until they are absent altogether in the distal part of the ileum. Thus, cross-hatching of the barium shadow in the area of bowel containing valvulae is seen (jejunum) and an uninterrupted ribbon of barium is seen where valvulae are absent in the distal ileum (Figure 4.31).

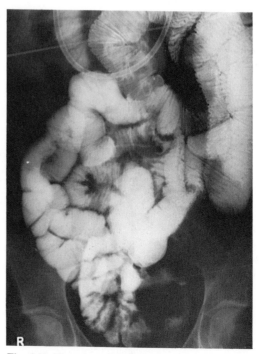

Fig. 4.31 Normal small bowel contrast enema.

CONGENITAL ABNORMALITIES

Meckel's diverticulum
This is rarely recognized as such in contrast examinations because it resembles a segment of normal bowel. A radionuclide scan may reveal its presence (see 'Radionuclide scan', page 107).

Malrotation
During development, the bowel normally rotates so that the large bowel becomes peripherally and the small bowel centrally placed. If normal rotation does not occur the large bowel lies on the left side and the small bowel on the right side of the abdomen.

Diverticula
In the erect position, fluid levels in the diverticula may be seen on plain films but are better demonstrated by barium examinations (Figure 4.32).

GRANULOMATA
The terminal ileum is the part of small bowel most frequently involved by granulomata, often with accompanying disease in the caecum. Three granulomata may occur:
1. Crohn's disease — common
2. Tuberculosis — rare
3. Actinomycosis — rare.

Crohn's Disease
In the earlier stages there is narrowing of the terminal ileum (string sign) and a nodular cobblestone pattern of the mucosa (Figure 4.33). As a result of spasm and later of fibrosis the caecum may not fill or may be irregular in contour. Later, fistulae between loops of bowel, or between bowel and bladder or vagina, may be demonstrable. If a significant length of small bowel is involved there may be normal segments of bowel between abnormal segments (skip lesions).

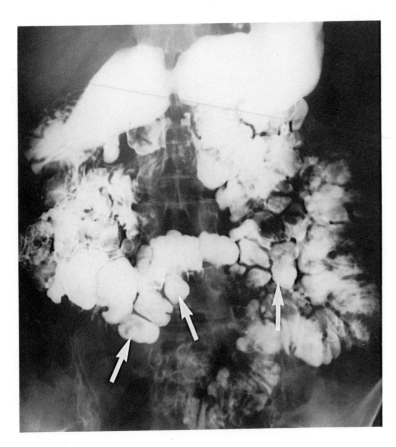

Fig. 4.32 Small intestinal diverticula (→) on barium meal and follow-through.

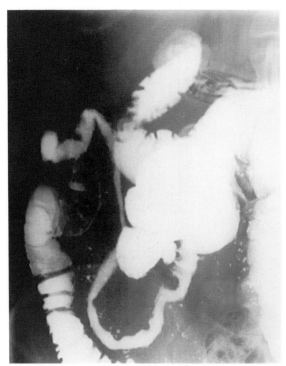

Fig. 4.33 Crohn's disease of terminal ileum showing 'string' sign.

Tuberculosis
In hyperplastic tuberculosis, the caecum and/or terminal ileum is found to be contracted, rigid and irregular. The appearances of the caecum are difficult to distinguish from actinomycosis or carcinoma, but evidence of tuberculosis elsewhere may be helpful in making a decision.

Actinomycosis
This is a rare condition presenting as a contracted and irregular caecum and terminal ileum, and is often indistinguishable from carcinoma or other granulomas. The diagnosis is made by mycology.

OBSTRUCTION
Erect and supine films of the abdomen must always be obtained in suspected small bowel obstruction.
The supine film will show gas-distended loops in which the valvulae conniventes can be clearly seen. The number of gas filled loops and the number of loops showing the presence or absence of valvulae will give an indication of the level of the obstruction (Figure 4.34). The erect

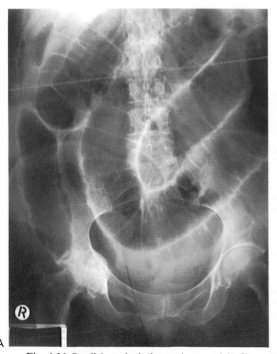
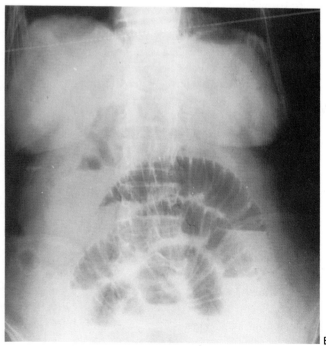

Fig. 4.34 Small intestinal obstruction on plain films. (A) Supine. (B) Erect.

film will show gas and fluid levels in the bowel, and again the number of fluid levels can help in determining the level of the obstruction. In very high obstructions there may be no fluid levels or distended loops because intestinal contents have been vomited.

It is important to realize that fluid levels and distended loops do not always indicate obstruction since they may also be seen in cases of adynamic ileus, and in electrolyte disturbances such as uraemia (pseudo-obstruction).

The fluid levels in small bowel obstruction tend to be short, 3–5 cm. The striations due to the valvulae conniventes run from one margin of the bowel completely across the gas-distended loop to the opposite margin to give the typical ladder pattern.

Small bowel loops and fluid levels may sometimes be seen in large bowel obstruction but a distended caecum, gas-filled colonic loops, and fluid levels in the large bowel will also be seen.

Differential diagnosis
Large bowel and small bowel obstruction are distinguished by the following criteria:

1. Fluid levels: short in small bowel — long in colon; often very numerous in small bowel.

2. Gas-filled loops: jejunal loops show ladder pattern, distal ileal loops have parallel walls. Colonic loops show haustration, except in the sigmoid colon which may resemble ileum.

Gastrograffin® or barium may be used if it is desired to outline the obstruction in small bowel, but barium by mouth should *never* be used in a suspected large bowel obstruction.

It is important to distinguish between acute obstruction, strangulation, and adynamic ileus; this is done by examination of the valvulae and of the distance between adjacent loops of distended bowel.

1. In acute obstruction the gas-filled loops are not separated by any significant space and the valvulae are well defined.

2. In strangulation the space between loops is increased and has a saw tooth shape. The valvulae are thickened.

3. In adynamic ileus there is an even increase in the space between loops and the valvulae are ill defined.

Gallstone ileus
In addition to the picture of small bowel obstruction there is evidence of gas in the biliary tree. The gallstone causing obstruction is often not seen because it may not be well calcified. The gas reaches the biliary tree via the fistula between the gall bladder and the duodenum at the site where the gallstone ulcerated through the walls of these structures.

MECONIUM ILEUS
This condition in the newborn is the result of fibrosis of the pancreas. Pancreatic enzymes cannot reach the bowel and the meconium becomes thick and plugs the bowel in the distal part of the ileum.

Radiological appearances
Gas-distended loops of small bowel with or without fluid levels are present and the mass of meconium can be seen in the pelvis and lower abdomen (Figure 4.35).

Meconium peritonitis
This is due to meconium escaping into the peritoneal cavity through a defect in the bowel wall. The meconium becomes encrusted with lime salts and this calcification can be seen on plain films of the abdomen (Figure 4.36). The condition has been recognized in pre-natal as well as in post-natal babies.

NEOPLASMS

Benign tumours
The common benign tumours are adenomata or lipomata and are usually only discovered when they lead to an intussusception.

Malignant tumours
Adenocarcinomata, although rare, are the most common type of malignancy; they produce a stricture of the bowel.

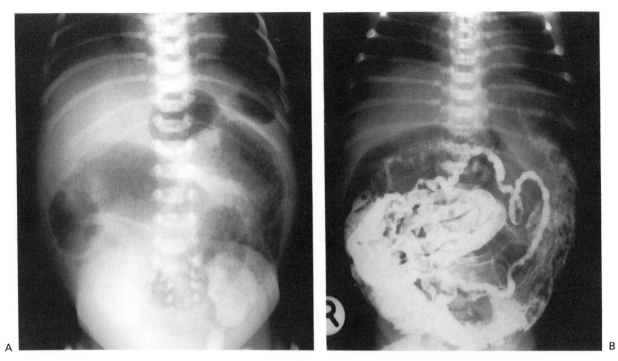

Fig. 4.35 (A) Meconium ileus on plain film of abdomen. (B) Contrast enema in meconium ileus, showing micro-colon.

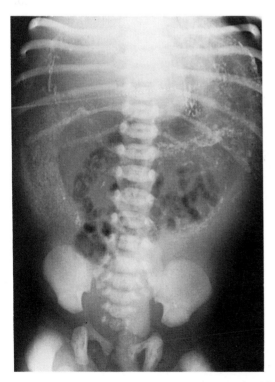

Fig. 4.36 Peritoneal calcification in meconium peritonitis.

INTUSSUSCEPTION

In this condition, which may affect small or large bowel or both, a segment of bowel (the intussusceptum) becomes invaginated into another segment (the intussuscipiens). In children the condition may develop without obvious cause, but in adults it is usually precipitated by the presence of a polyp.

Radiological appearances

1. Plain radiographs may reveal a soft tissue mass in the abdomen, gas-distended coils of bowel, and fluid levels due to obstruction.

2. In cases involving the colon a barium enema may show (Figure 4.37): (a) obstruction to the flow of barium with a concave filling defect at the head of the barium column; (b) a small amount of barium entering the narrow lumen of the involved bowel; (c) Barium may enter the space between the intussusceptum and the intussuscipiens and produce a coiled spring appearance.

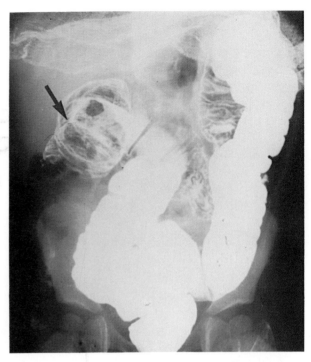

Fig. 4.37 Ileo-caecal intussusception showing 'coil-spring' appearance (→).

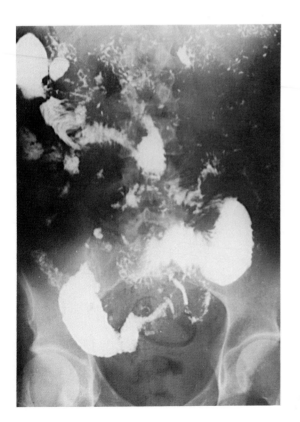

MALABSORPTION

There are multiple causes of malabsorption and the reader is referred to a medical text for a complete list. A barium meal follow-through examination shows several changes.

Radiological appearances (Figure 4.38)

1. Flocculation of the barium.

2. Segmentation of the barium column in the small bowel with areas of dilatation.

3. Usually delayed progress of the barium but sometimes rapid progress.

4. Dilution of the barium in the distal small bowel.

5. Coarse mucosal pattern.

Fig. 4.38 Barium follow-through in malabsorption, showing flocculation and segmentation of the barium column.

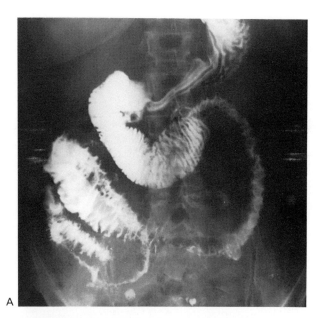

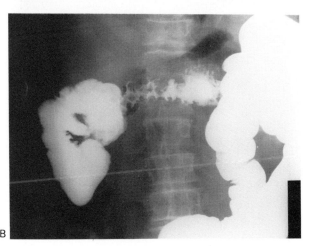

VASCULAR LESIONS

The radiological appearances of occlusion of the vascular supply to the small bowel depend on the vessel affected. The occlusion may be sudden as with thrombosis or embolism or may develop slowly as in atherosclerosis.

Acute arterial occlusion

This leads to ileus, with multiple fluid levels and gas distended loops. If the superior mesenteric artery is involved at its origin the right half of the large bowel also shows gas distension and fluid levels.

Mesenteric venous thrombosis

This leads to a distorted loop, or loops of small bowel with 'finger-print' filling defects in the barium due to haemorrhage into the bowel wall (Figure 4.39a).

Ischaemia

This usually involves the distal transverse and descending colon, at the junction of the blood supply from the inferior and superior mesenteric arteries. Plain films show the appearances of obstruction, with oedema of the mucosa in the affected segment. This may be more clearly demonstrated by barium enema (Figure 4.39b). If natural resolution occurs, a long smooth stricture may develop. Angiography of the supplying arteries may demonstrate stenosis or obstruction.

Fig. 4.39 (A) Barium meal showing haemorrhage into wall of small bowel.
(B) Barium enema in ischaemic colitis showing narrow area in transverse colon.

The large bowel

METHODS OF INVESTIGATION

Plain radiographs
Erect and supine films of the abdomen are useful in cases of suspected obstruction.

Air contrast enema
This has largely replaced the ordinary barium enema. A small quantity of barium sulphate suspension is instilled into the colon *per rectum* and then air is blown into the colon to distend it. The patient is rotated during the procedure so that the walls of the colon are coated with a thin film of barium.

LESIONS OF THE COLON

Congenital abnormalities

Malrotation
This has been considered in the section on small bowel (see page 108).

Imperforate anus
Plain films will demonstrate the situation. The examination is not performed for several hours after birth (six is recommended) to allow swallowed air to reach the rectum. A metal marker is placed on the skin at the site where the anus should be, the infant is then inverted and films are made with the child in this position. The films reveal the distance between the metal marker and the gas in the rectum (Figure 4.40).

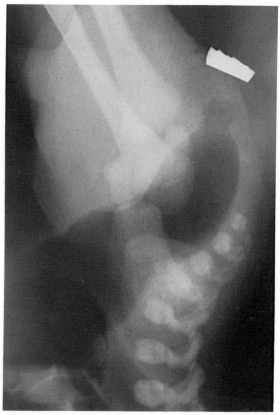

Fig. 4.40 Inverted film in imperforate anus. The gas shows the extent of the rectum, and the skin marker is in the anal dimple.

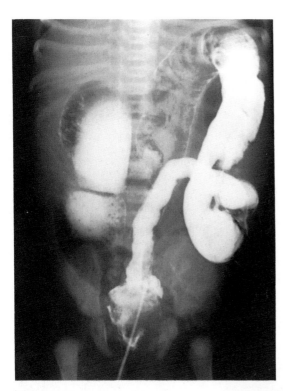

Fig. 4.41 Hirschsprung's disease of colon. The long narrow segment is well shown on contrast enema.

Hirschsprung's disease
There is an absence of ganglion cells in the myenteric nerve plexuses in a segment of bowel usually just above the anus, leading to an area of smooth narrowing of the bowel at this site. Above this the bowel is markedly dilated and filled with faeces (Figure 4.41).

ULCERATIVE COLITIS

Acute phase
1. A plain film may show a markedly gas distended colon with no fluid levels — *toxic dilatation.*
2. The sharp definition of the edge of the barium coating the colonic wall is lost and the margin becomes granular due to multiple small superficial ulcers.
3. Later there may be hypertrophy of the mucosa between the ulcers to give a pseudo-polyposis (Figure 4.42).

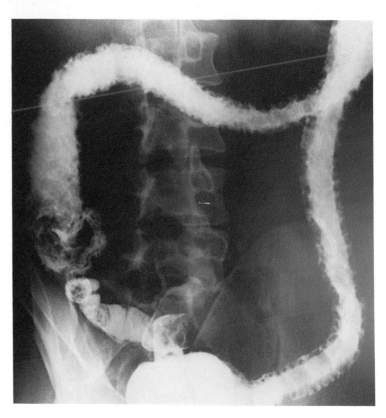

Fig. 4.42 Ulcerative colitis. Active stage with pseudopolyps shown by barium enema.

Chronic phase (Figure 4.43)

1. Mucosal pattern is lost and the colon becomes smooth.

2. The portion of the colon involved becomes narrowed and haustration is lost.

3. Shortening of the colon occurs and this with the smooth narrowing and absence of haustration gives the 'pipe stem colon'.

Ulcerative colitis tends to start in the rectum as a proctitis and then extends back along the colon in a continuous fashion — there are no skip areas.

CROHN'S DISEASE

Radiological appearances
The following features are seen in a barium enema (Figure 4.44).

1. Irregular narrowing of segments of bowel which usually involve the whole circumference but which may only involve part of the circumference. There is a gradual transition from normal to involved bowel.

2. Rose thorn ulcers. The ulceration in Crohn's disease is deep and linear and barium entering these ulcers produces rose thorn shaped projections from the bowel.

3. Skip lesions. There are frequently segments of uninvolved bowel separating segments which are involved by the disease.

4. The rectum tends to be involved in a minority of cases but perianal changes are common.

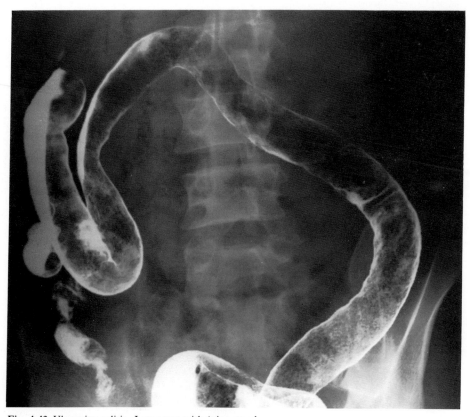

Fig. 4.43 Ulcerative colitis. Late stage with 'pipe-stem' appearance.

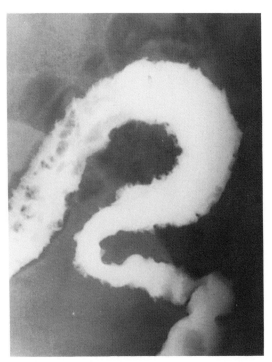

Fig. 4.44 Active Crohn's disease of colon, with 'rose-thorn' ulcers.

ISCHAEMIC COLITIS

As the result of impairment of blood supply, which is not sufficient to produce death and gangrene, there is oedema of the bowel wall and haemorrhage into the wall which produce smooth filling defects (thumb-printing) in the barium along the margin of the affected segment, which is also narrowed (see Figure 4.39). It is not uncommon to find these changes in the region of a carcinoma.

DIVERTICULAR DISEASE

The diverticula have narrow necks, are rounded, multiple and most common in the sigmoid colon (Figure 4.45). If faeces are present in the diverticula the filling with barium will be incomplete and will give crescentic shadows. There is marked irregularity and narrowing of the bowel wall in the area of the diverticula in some cases and there may also be

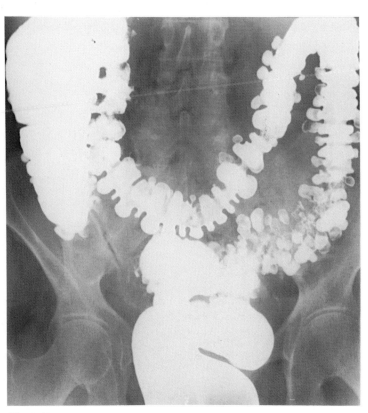

Fig. 4.45 Diverticulosis of colon.

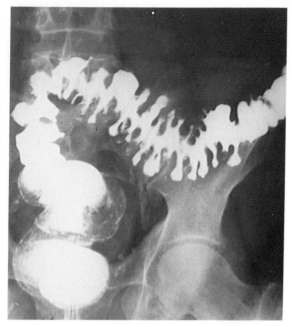

Fig. 4.46 Diverticulitis of sigmoid colon, with lumenal narrowing.

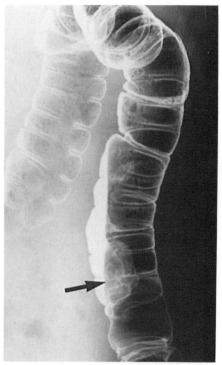

Fig. 4.47 Polyp (→) in descending colon. Double contrast enema.

some shortening of the segment involved (Figure 4.46). In the later stage of the disease fistulae may form between the bowel and bladder, or between large and small bowel. These are not readily shown radiologically.

NEOPLASMS

Benign tumours
These may appear in the barium enema as smooth, round, filling defects often with a pedicle (Figure 4.47). In familial polyposis there are multiple smooth, round, filling defects (Figure 4.48). Malignant change in these polyps is seen as thickening of the adjacent bowel wall and irregularity of the pedicle of the polyp.

Malignant tumours
Carcinoma is by far the most common malignant tumour and occurs in two main forms, encephaloid and scirrhous.

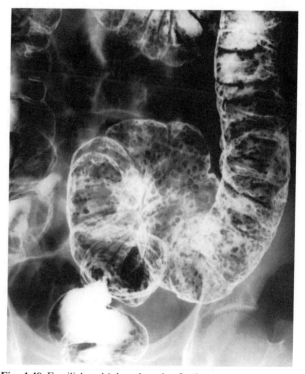

Fig. 4.48 Familial multiple polyposis of colon.

Encephaloid tumours
The feature is an irregular filling defect in the barium (Figure 4.49).

Scirrhous tumours
The features are:

1. A segment of irregular narrowing with shoulder defects at each end of the stricture — apple core appearance (Figure 4.50)

2. There may be signs of obstruction proximal to the site of the lesion.

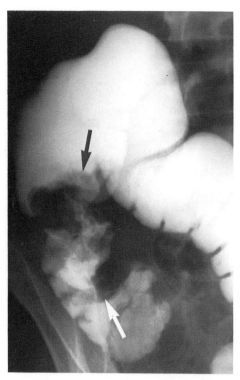

Fig. 4.49 Encephaloid (fungating) carcinoma of colon (→).

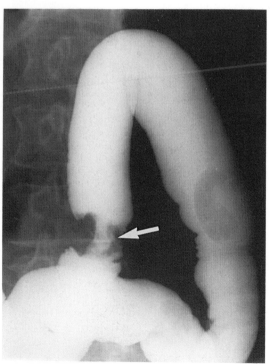

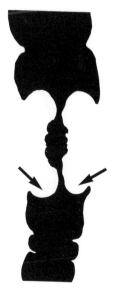

Fig. 4.50 (A) 'Ring' carcinoma of colon (→).
(B) Diagram of 'ring' carcinoma, showing 'shoulders' (→).

OBSTRUCTION

Radiological appearances

1. Plain radiographs: *Erect and supine films are essential*. The erect film will show long fluid levels in the bowel. The supine film will show gas-distended loops of large bowel with the typical haustrated margins (Figure 4.51).

2. Contrast enema: the cause of the obstruction will be outlined, e.g. a malignant stricture.

Sigmoid volvulus

Radiological appearances

1. Plain radiographs: a huge, distended, gas-filled loop of sigmoid colon is seen passing from the pelvis up into the abdomen. There may be a long fluid level within the loop.

2. Contrast enema: this shows obstruction to the flow of barium at the site of the twist and at that site the barium in the colon has the shape of an eagle's beak.

A

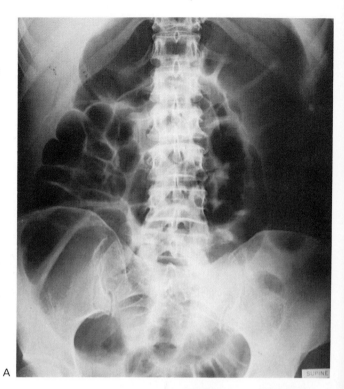

B

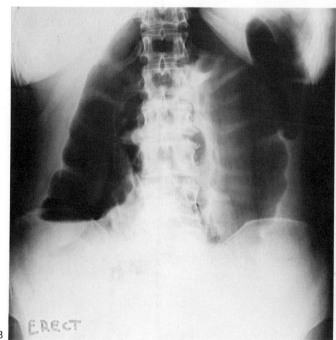

Fig. 4.51 Large bowel obstruction shown on plain abdominal films.

(A) Supine, showing distension.
(B) Erect, showing fluid levels.

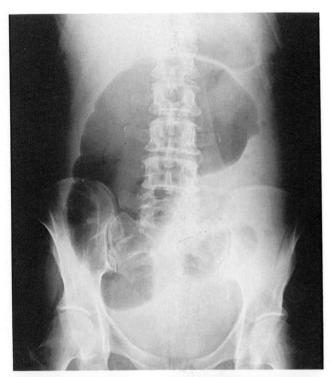

A

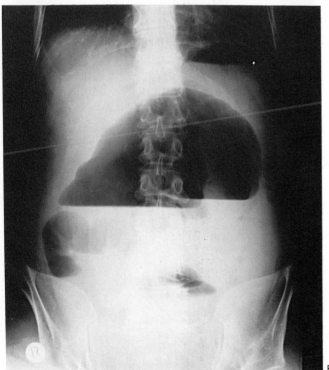

B

Caecal volvulus

Radiological appearances
Plain radiographs: these show a very large gas-distended loop of colon lying either to the right of the midline or in the central abdomen. There is usually a long fluid level present in the loop if the film is made with the patient erect (Figure 4.52).

Fig. 4.52 Caecal volvulus, shown on plain films of abdomen.
(A) Supine, showing grossly distended loop.
(B) Erect, with long fluid level.

GAS CYSTS (PNEUMATOSIS COLI)

Radiological appearances
1. Plain radiographs: oval or rounded areas of radiolucency are seen along the margin of the colon.
2. Contrast enema: (a) areas of radiolucency bordering the barium column in the bowel; (b) Crescentic smooth filling defects along the margin of the barium column due to the gas cysts impinging on the lumen of the bowel (Figure 4.53).

MEGACOLON
There is marked dilatation of the colon *and rectum*, which are usually loaded with faeces, but there is no narrow segment as in Hirschsprung's disease.

MELAENA OR BRIGHT BLOOD LOSS PR
Melaena or bright blood loss from the large bowel may arise from colonic lesions as well as resulting from upper gastrointestinal pathology. A suggested sequence of imaging examinations for these signs is outlined in Diagnostic decision tree 4, page 303.

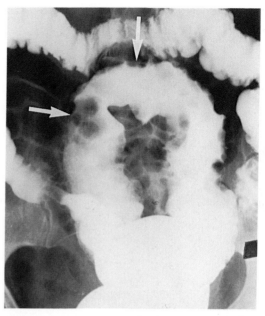

Fig. 4.53 Pneumatosis coli, showing gas cysts in colon wall (→).

Diaphragmatic herniae

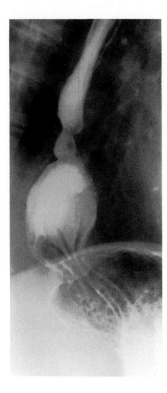

Fig. 4.54 Sliding hiatus hernia, with stricture, shown by barium swallow.

HIATUS HERNIA

The oesophagus passes through the fibres of the right crus of the diaphragm to reach the abdomen and enter the stomach. If for some reason, such as the deposition of fat between the fibres of the crus, the oesophageal hiatus in the diaphragm becomes weakened and stretched, the stomach can protrude up through the hiatus to produce an hiatus hernia (Figure 4.54).

There are three types of hiatus hernia (Figure 4.55):

1. Sliding hiatus hernia: the portion of stomach containing the gastro-oesophageal junction passes up through the hiatus.

2. Rolling hiatus hernia (para-oesophageal hernia): the fundus of the stomach passes up through the hiatus and lies to the left lateral side of the lower oesophagus and the oesophago-gastric junction remains beneath the diaphragm.

3. Mixed sliding and rolling hiatus hernia. Three mechanisms have been suggested as the

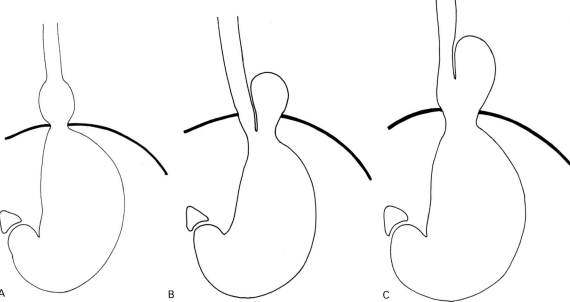

Fig. 4.55 Diagrams showing types of oesophageal hiatus hernia.
(A) Sliding. (B) Para-oesophageal. (C) Combined sliding and para-oesophageal.

reason that gastro-oesophageal reflux does not normally occur: (a) the fibres of the right crus of the diaphragm compress the lower end of the oesophagus; (b) the acute angle of entry of the oesophagus into the stomach; (c) a physiological sphincter at the lower end of the oesophagus.

When an hiatus hernia is present these mechanisms break down with reflux of acid gastric contents into the oesophagus, producing oesophagitis which may go on to ulceration, fibrosis and stricture formation. If there is ectopic, gastric-type mucosa in the oesphagus a true peptic ulcer, with or without stricture formation, may occur (see Figure 4.11).

FORAMEN OF MORGAGNI HERNIA

The foramen is situated anteriorly where there may be a gap in the muscular attachment of the diaphragm to the xiphisternum. Through this, omentum or transverse colon may protrude. The radiological appearances are those of an area of opacity or gas-containing loops of bowel in the angle between the heart and the right hemidiaphragm (Figure 4.56).

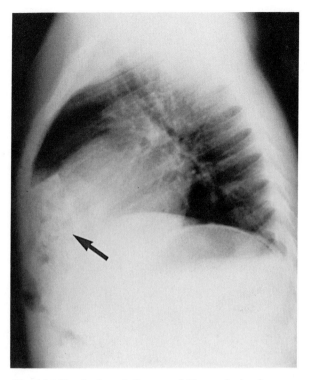

Fig. 4.56 Hernia through foramen of Morgagni, showing gas-containing gut in anterior mediastinum (→).

FORAMEN OF BOCHDALEK HERNIA

This foramen sometimes occurs posteriorly in the diaphragm at the site of the pleuro-peritoneal canals. Abdominal contents such as bowel, spleen and kidney may all herniate through the foramen and can be seen either as gas- containing coils or as a solid mass in the chest in the para-vertebral area just above the diaphragm posteriorly.

TRAUMATIC HERNIA

Rupture of the diaphragm may allow abdominal contents to enter the thorax. It occurs most commonly on the left side. The condition must be distinguished from marked elevation of the dome of the diaphragm, as in eventration. Eventration is the term used for a high, immobile hemidiaphragm resulting from poor diaphragmatic muscle development. In eventration the diaphragm reaches the chest wall anteriorly, laterally and posteriorly, but the shadow of the gas-containing stomach which has become displaced upwards through a traumatic hernia may not reach the chest wall at all these points.

Plain radiographs in the acute abdomen

Plain films can be of great value in the diagnosis of the acute abdomen. Contrast studies, particularly of the biliary and urinary tracts, may give additional information.

INTESTINAL OBSTRUCTION
Supine and erect films may show gas-distended loops and fluid levels and, in the case of gallstone ileus, gas will be seen in the biliary tree. (Details of the appearances are given in the sections on small and large bowel, pages 109 and 120.)

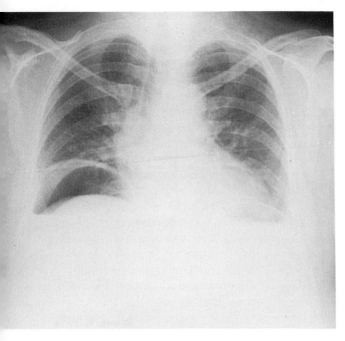

Fig. 4.57 Erect radiograph of chest showing free sub-diaphragmatic gas due to ruptured viscus.

PERFORATION OF THE GASTROINTESTINAL TRACT
Peptic ulcer is the common cause but perforation of colonic diverticula and in association with neoplasms occurs.

Radiological signs
1. Free gas in the peritoneal cavity. This is seen in approximately 80% of perforated peptic ulcers. The gas collects in the highest part of the peritoneal cavity and is seen beneath the diaphragm with the patient erect (Figure 4.57) or under the lateral wall of the abdomen with the patient in the lateral decubitus position. Gas under the left dome of the diaphragm may be difficult to distinguish from gas in the fundus of the stomach, but it is readily seen under the right dome. For practical purposes gas under the right dome is always abnormal since bowel rarely interposes between liver and diaphragm.
2. Localized collections of gas in the pelvis. These may be seen in colonic diverticular perforation and are due to gas-producing organisms in an abscess.
3. Water-soluble contrast medium may be seen to escape into the peritoneal cavity through a perforated peptic ulcer.

CHOLECYSTITIS
There are no direct signs on plain films unless opaque stones are visible (only 20% of gallstones are radio-opaque), or gas can be seen in the gall bladder wall or cavity. The indirect sign is a localized ileus of bowel in the area (sentinel loop).

Obstructive and non-obstructive cholecystitis may be differentiated by intravenous cholangiography, providing there is no jaundice, when contrast enters the gall bladder in the non-obstructive form. In obstructed cases ultrasound is useful in showing calculi and changes in the gall bladder wall.

ACUTE APPENDICITIS AND ACUTE SALPINGITIS

These give no direct signs but there may be a sentinel loop in the area.

ACUTE PANCREATITIS

Plain radiographs may show:
1. No abnormality
2. A localized small bowel ileus in the area
3. Absence of gas in the transverse colon
4. A fluid level in the lesser sac due to abscess formation.

PERINEPHRIC ABSCESS

Plain radiographs may show:
1. Obliteration of the renal outline
2. Partial obliteration of the psoas shadow.

SUBPHRENIC ABSCESS

Although not usually presenting as an acute abdomen it is best dealt with in this section and may show (Figure 4.58):
1. Elevation and reduced excursion of a dome of the diaphragm
2. If gas-producing organisms are present, gas, usually in the form of globules, will be seen beneath the diaphragm
3. A small pleural effusion
4. Localized inflammatory change in the base of the adjacent lung.

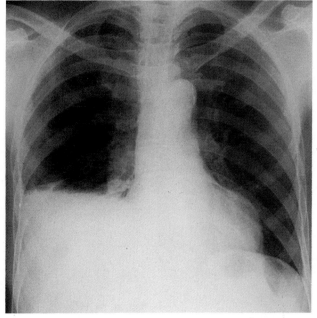

Fig. 4.58 Right subphrenic abscess producing elevation of right hemidiaphragm and a small pleural effusion.

CALCULI

Calculi may be seen in the biliary or urinary tracts. Intravenous pyelography may be useful with suspected ureteric calculus by showing delay in excretion of contrast by the kidney on that side, and later by contrast filling the system down to the site of the calculus. Intravenous cholangiography will demonstrate stones in the bile duct and cholecystography will show calculi in the gall bladder providing there is no jaundice. Ultrasound may show stones in the gall bladder or ducts even when jaundice is present.

MESENTERIC VASCULAR LESIONS

Mesenteric occlusion, arterial or venous (see small bowel section, page 113).

AORTIC ANEURYSM

(See vascular section, page 79.) An expanding aneurysm may be painful and if it leaks, either into the surrounding retroperitoneal tissues or subintimally (dissecting aneurysm), it produces an acute abdominal emergency. Plain films may show a mass, loss of psoas shadows, and ileus. Computerized tomography and angiography will show the dilatation and leak, if necessary, prior to emergency surgery.

5 Liver, Spleen, Biliary Tract and Pancreas

The liver and spleen

METHODS OF INVESTIGATION

Plain radiographs
The presence of calcification is shown, e.g. a calcified hydatid in the liver or opaque gallstones may be seen (Figure 5.1).

Computerized tomography
This will delineate abnormal densities such as cysts, haematomas and some tumours.

Ultrasound
This allows assessment of the presence and nature of space-occupying lesions such as cysts and tumours (Figure 5.2).

Radionuclide scanning
The radiopharmaceutical, a colloid material, is injected intravenously and taken up by the Kupffer cells in the liver but is not concentrated by abnormal hepatic and splenic tissue, which thus produce 'cold spots' (absence of radioactivity) on the scan. These cold spots are, however, not definitive of any specific pathology.

Angiography
This demonstrates the arterial and/or venous aspects of liver and spleen. It is performed by percutaneous catheterization of the appropriate arteries (hepatic, splenic or branch vessels) or veins, from a femoral puncture and injection of contrast medium.

Splenoportography
Contrast medium is injected directly into the spleen percutaneously. The medium enters and fills the splenic vein and portal venous system. This investigation is now rarely used except where demonstration of a shunt such as a porto-caval anastomosis is required.

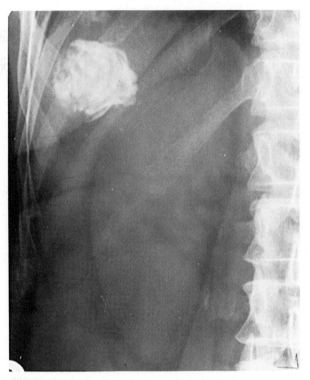

Fig. 5.1 Calcified hydatid in liver. Plain radiograph.

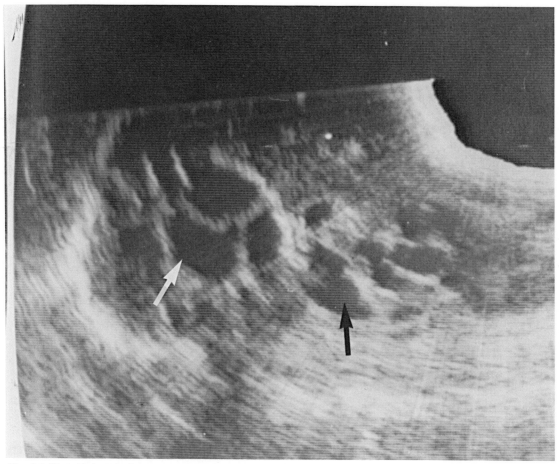

Fig. 5.2 Hydatid cysts in liver on ultrasound (→).

LESIONS OF THE LIVER

CONGENITAL ABNORMALITIES

The liver varies remarkably in shape and size, depending on habitus. Congenital cystic disease, sometimes associated with renal cystic disease, is easily demonstrated by CT, nuclear medicine and ultrasound.

TRAUMA

Tears or contusion of the liver may sometimes be present with few clinical signs other than unexplained blood loss. Radionuclide scanning or CT will demonstrate or exclude damage to the liver or spleen. Ultrasound is also useful for demonstrating perihepatic and perisplenic collections. In continuing haemorrhage angiography may be used to demonstrate the bleeding point and permit trans-catheter embolization of the bleeding vessel.

NEOPLASMS

Metastatic deposits
Radionuclide scanning (Figure 5.3) and
ultrasound used in combination have a 90%
accuracy in showing metastases, whereas
individually they have an accuracy of only 75%.
Computerized tomography is usually reserved for
elucidation of cases which remain as problems
following radionuclide scanning and ultrasound.

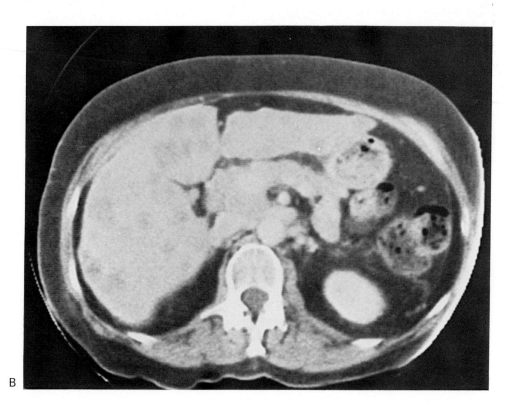

STATIC LIVER STUDY

ANT./MARKER   ANTERIOR

RT   LT

30° LT. ANT. OBLIQUE   POSTERIOR

RT   LT   RT

RT. LATERAL

P   A

A   DOSE: 2mCi of ^{99m}TC S/C, given I.V.

Fig. 5.3 Tumour metastases in
liver demonstrated by:
(A) radionuclide scan using
sulphur colloid, (B) CT scan,
(C) ultrasound.

B

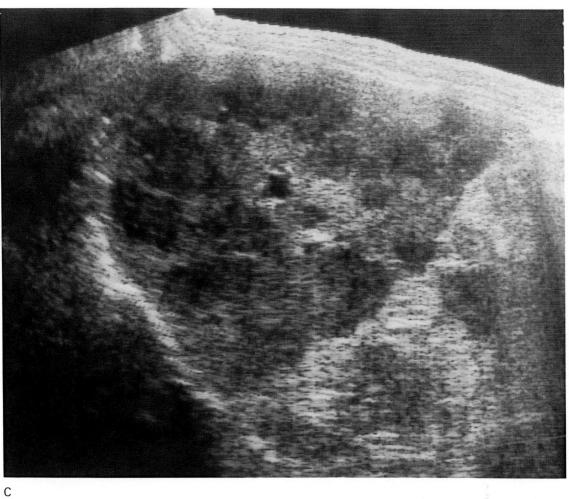

C

Primary malignant tumours
Usually a hepatoma, it may be unicentric or
multicentric. The same sequence of tests is used
as with metastases (Figure 5.4). In both primary
and metastatic deposits radiologically guided
biopsy may be used for a definitive diagnosis.

Benign tumours
The adenoma, which is the least rare, may occur
after the use of oral contraceptives. It shows
normal or exaggerated uptake on radionuclide
scanning, solidity on ultrasound, and
hypervascularity on angiography.

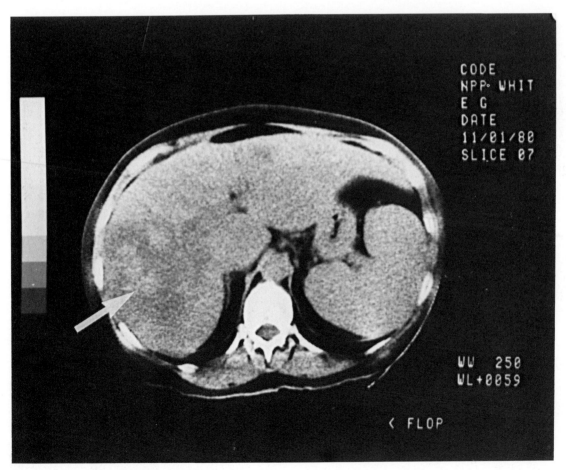

Fig. 5.4 Hepatoma shown on CT scan (→).

INFLAMMATORY LESIONS

Acute
The localized form is the liver abscess, usually either amoebic or pyogenic. There may be liver enlargement or gas in the abscess, on plain films. Nuclear medicine scanning, computerized tomography (Figure 5.5), and ultrasound all show the lesion well, ultrasound often showing the fluid or semi-fluid nature of the contents.

Chronic
Usually viral or auto-immune in nature. Plain films show initially a large and often later a small liver. Computerized tomography and ultrasound are non-specific.

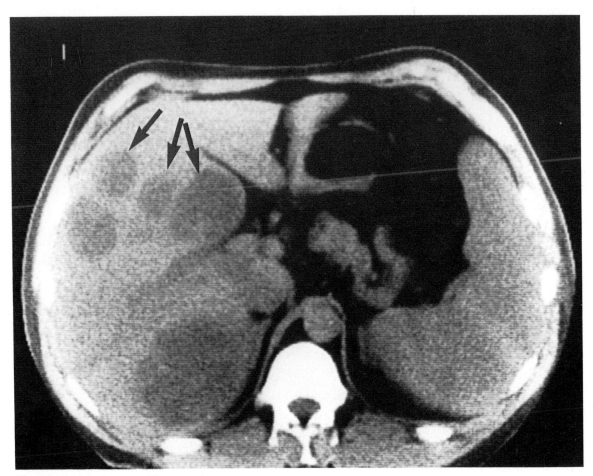

Fig. 5.5 Multiple abscesses of liver (→); CT scan.

Cirrhosis
This is the late stage of inflammatory or degenerative liver disease, with fine or coarse scarring. Imaging may show initially a large and later a small liver, with reduced hepatocellular function. The size, shape and general density are shown on all imaging systems, but nuclear medicine is particularly useful in demonstrating the reduced function (Fig. 5.6). Biopsy is required for histological characterization.

PORTAL HYPERTENSION
This may complicate cirrhosis or hepatic vein obstruction with, in some cases, the development of porto-systemic varices. Bleeding from oesophageal varices may be life-threatening. The site and size of the shunting and varices may be shown by splenoportography (Figure 5.7), or arteriography of the coeliac and mesenteric arteries, with late venous views.

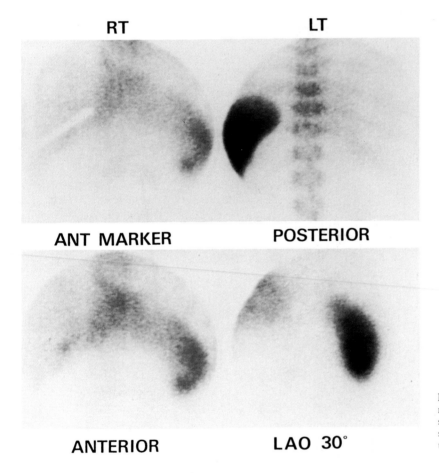

Fig. 5.6 Cirrhosis of liver on radionuclide sulphur colloid scan, showing low liver uptake, large spleen and high bone marrow uptake.

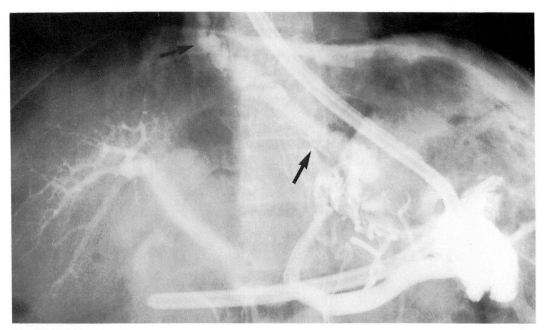

Fig. 5.7 Percutaneous splenoportogram, showing shunting through oesophageal varices (→). There is a naso-gastric tube in the stomach.

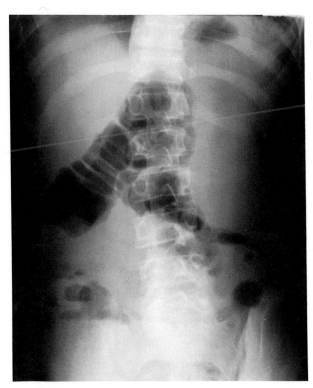

Fig. 5.8 Erect radiograph of abdomen in case of ruptured spleen, showing medial displacement of splenic flexure of colon.

LESIONS OF THE SPLEEN

The spleen is essentially a component of the lympho-reticular system, but its upper abdominal position and involvement with the hepatoportal vascular system renders some consideration here appropriate.

CONGENITAL ABNORMALITIES
Absence is rare, but is important to note in neonates as it may be associated with complex cardiac defects. Polysplenia is also rare.

TRAUMA
Splenic rupture is a surgical emergency. Plain films may be normal, or show signs of local trauma, such as rib fractures. Displacement of the stomach or splenic flexure of the colon downwards or medially indicates the presence of a perisplenic haematoma (Figure 5.8).

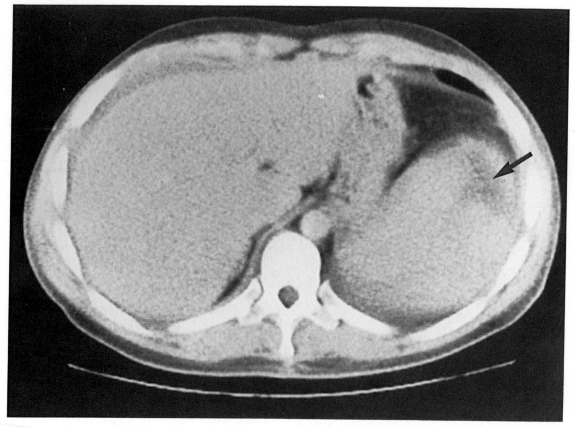

Fig. 5.9 Subcapsular haematoma of spleen (→) shown by CT.

Computerized tomography and ultrasound will show a perisplenic, and sometimes an intrasplenic, haematoma (Figure 5.9); nuclear medicine, although probably less accurate in showing perisplenic collections, shows the splenic rupture rather better. Non-traumatic follow-up of splenic injury has shown that many ruptures heal spontaneously so that splenectomy, with its attendant complications, is now necessary only for strict surgical indications such as continuing bleeding.

NEOPLASM
Neoplastic involvement of the spleen is rare, other than in the lymphomas, which frequently present with splenomegaly.

INFLAMMATORY
Pyogenic abscesses are rare, show as splenomegaly on plain radiography, and are clearly seen on CT, ultrasound and nuclear medicine. Calcification in healed abscesses may be seen on plain films.

SPLENOMEGALY
This is a common presenting sign in a wide spectrum of diseases such as lymphomas, haemolytic anaemias, portal hypertension, amyloid and lipid storage disease, as well as malnutrition. Although imaging techniques display splenomegaly they do not indicate the specific cause. Histological, haematological and biochemical tests are required to ascertain the aetiology. (See page 85.)

Biliary tract

Methods of investigation

Plain radiographs

Twenty per cent of biliary calculi contain calcium and are therefore visible on plain films (radio-opaque calculi) Figure 5.10). Gas in the bile ducts or wall of the gallbladder is visible on plain films. Gas in the bile ducts usually results from operations on the ampulla of Vater, or from fistula formation following ulceration of a calculus from the gall bladder through to the duodenum. Gas in the gall bladder wall occurs in emphysematous cholecystitis.

Ultrasound

This will demonstrate changes in the gall bladder wall in cholecystitis, the presence or absence of calculi in the ducts or gall bladder, and whether the ducts are normal or dilated.

Benefits of ultrasound

1. In cases of jaundice the state of the duct system will indicate whether the jaundice is obstructive or hepato-cellular.

2. It gives information about the state of the gall bladder when it is non-functioning on oral cholecystography.

3. It indicates the presence or absence of calculi in the biliary tract in cases of jaundice or where there is a non-functioning gall bladder on oral cholecystography.

4. The patient receives no radiation.

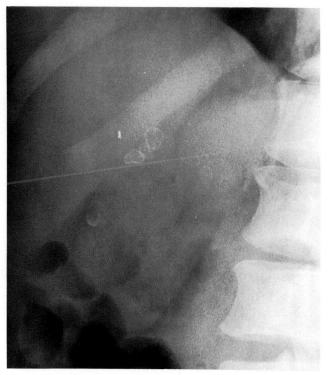

Fig. 5.10 Calcified gallstones on plain radiograph.

Oral cholecystography

Contrast medium taken orally is absorbed from the small bowel, excreted by the liver, and concentrated in the gall bladder, resulting in opacification of the gall bladder (Figure 5.11). **NB** A plain film of the gall bladder area must precede oral cholecystography because the contrast medium may obscure opaque calculi. Radiolucent (non-calcium containing) calculi show as filling defects in the contrast medium. Non-opacification of the gall bladder usually denotes gall bladder disease, perhaps with obstruction of the cystic duct by a gallstone.

Contraindications
Jaundice and liver failure — the liver will not excrete the contrast medium.

Intravenous cholangiography

Contrast medium given intravenously is excreted by the liver and opacifies the bile ducts. Calculi in the ducts are recognized as filling defects in the contrast medium. The ducts can be opacified even when the gall bladder has been removed.

Contraindications
1. Jaundice and liver failure — the medium is not excreted.
2. Oral cholecystography and intravenous cholangiography examinations should be separated by a week because of the increased toxicity from the combination of the two media.

Operative cholangiography

Contrast medium is injected directly into the duct system at operation. Calculi and stenotic lesions of the ducts may be demonstrated.

Postoperative cholangiography

Contrast medium is instilled into the duct system via a T-tube which has been placed *in situ* at operation. Retained calculi may be demonstrated and the presence or absence of free drainage of the duct into the duodenum shown (Figure 5.12).

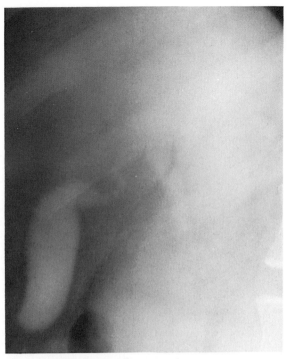

Fig. 5.11 Normal oral cholecystogram.

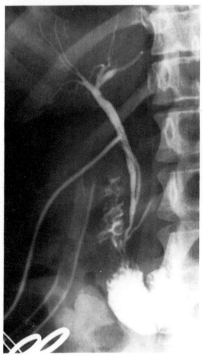

Fig. 5.12 Post-operative T-tube cholangiogram. There are no residual calculi, and contrast flows freely into the duodenum.

ERCP (Endoscopic retrograde catheterization of the pancreatic and/or bile ducts)

The bile and/or pancreatic ducts are catheterized via a gastroduodenoscope and contrast medium injected. The main use is the demonstration of the site of duct obstruction.

PTC (Percutaneous transhepatic cholangiography)

This is used in cases of obstructive jaundice to demonstrate the site of obstruction from above. A long thin needle is passed through the skin and peritoneum into the liver to enter a bile duct into which contrast medium is injected. In a modification of this procedure the bile ducts may be catheterized to allow external drainage of the obstructed ducts or a stent may be passed through a stenosis to permit internal drainage.

LESIONS OF THE BILIARY TRACT

CONGENITAL ATRESIA OF THE BILE DUCTS

Ultrasound or percutaneous transhepatic cholangiography will show the extent of the duct system.

NEOPLASMS

Carcinoma of the gall bladder

Filling of the gall bladder with contrast medium by oral cholecystography or intravenous cholangiography may show irregularity of the gall bladder wall. Ultrasound or computerized tomography may demonstrate a mass.

Neoplasms of bile ducts

These may be either: (1) intrahepatic and often multicentric, appearing on ultrasound, computerized tomography and a radionuclide scan as single or multiple space-occupying lesions, and on percutaneous transhepatic cholangiography or endoscopic retrograde cholangiography as strictures of the ducts; or (2) extrahepatic — ultrasound will show dilated ducts above the lesion but the diagnosis is usually made by PTC or ERCP (Figure 5.13).

Benign tumours

These are usually papillomata of the gall bladder which closely resemble calculi on oral cholecystography or ultrasound.

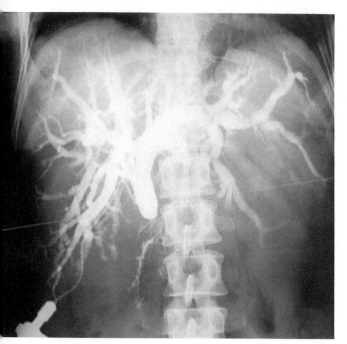

Fig. 5.13 Percutaneous transhepatic cholangiogram, showing obstruction of the common bile duct.

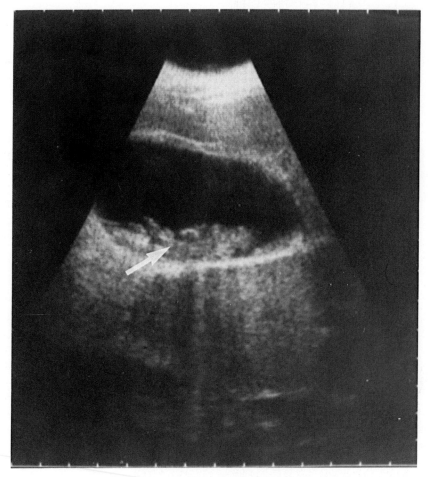

Fig. 5.14 Ultrasound of gall bladder containing calculi (→).

CHOLECYSTITIS

Acute cholecystitis
This is a surgical emergency but investigations, if necessary, include the following:

1. *Plain radiographs* may show a mass, opaque calculi, or gas in the lumen or wall of the gall bladder when there is gangrene with gas-forming organisms present.

2. *Ultrasound* may show a dilated, sometimes thick-walled, gall bladder and calculi if present (Figure 5.14).

3. *Intravenous cholangiography* or HIDA radionuclide scanning (Figure 5.15) will show duct patency and the presence or absence of calculi.

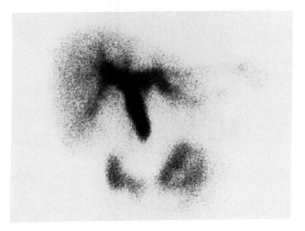

Fig. 5.15 Radionuclide HIDA scan, showing patency of bile ducts, but absence of filling of gall bladder due to acute cholecystitis. Common bile duct (→).

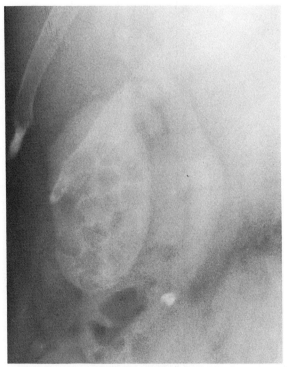

Fig. 5.16 Oral cholecystogram showing radiolucent calculi in the gall bladder, and a calcified calculus at the lower end of the common bile duct.

Chronic cholecystitis
This may require a battery of tests which, in order of preference, comprise the following:

1. Ultrasound may show the size and shape of the gall bladder, wall thickness, the presence or absence of calculi, and the state of the duct system.

2. Oral cholecystography may show the presence or absence of calculi and often poor concentration of contrast medium in the gall bladder (Figure 5.16).

3. If oral cholecystography fails to show the gall bladder or ducts, intravenous cholangiography will demonstrate the ducts and any contained calculi (Figure 5.17).

BILIARY CALCULI

Calculi in the gall bladder may be shown on plain films if radio-opaque (20%), by oral cholecystography if radiolucent, or in either case by ultrasound. Calculi in the duct system may be shown pre-operatively by ultrasound or intravenous cholangiography, at operation by operative cholangiography, and postoperatively by T-tube cholangiography or ERCP.

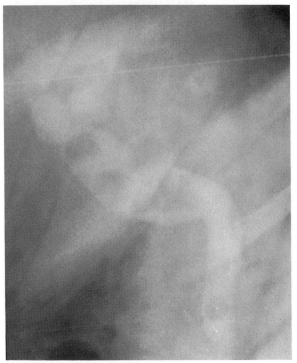

Fig. 5.17 Intravenous cholangiogram showing multiple radiolucent calculi in the dilated common bile duct.

CHOLANGITIS

Acute
Gas may occasionally be seen in the ducts or in a liver abscess on plain films.

Chronic
Strictures of the ducts may occur and are best shown by percutaneous transhepatic cholangiography or endoscopic retrograde cholangiography (See Fig. 5.13)

JAUNDICE

This is a sign common to many biliary tract and liver diseases and often presents diagnostic difficulty. Oral cholecystography and intravenous cholangiography are useless in the presence of jaundice because the contrast medium is not excreted by the liver.

Ultrasound will demonstrate with accuracy in excess of 90% any dilatation of bile ducts (Figure 5.18), the gall bladder and its state, and the level of obstruction if present. It may also show the presence of calculi or a pancreatic mass as the cause of the jaundice.

Computerized tomography with intravenous contrast medium reinforcement is equally as sensitive, but is slower and more expensive. Endoscopic retrograde cholangiography or pancreatography is useful in cases where ultrasound or computerized tomography have not shown the site and cause of an obstruction. ERCP has to a large extent replaced PTC, which is more invasive and carries higher risks to the patient.

PTC, by the introduction of an indwelling drainage catheter or internal stent, permits time for patient improvement before surgery or even obviates the need for a by-pass operation, especially in malignant disease (Figure 5.19).

The investigations needed for a patient with jaundice vary according to the cause and an appropriate sequence of the investigations is suggested in Table 5.1.

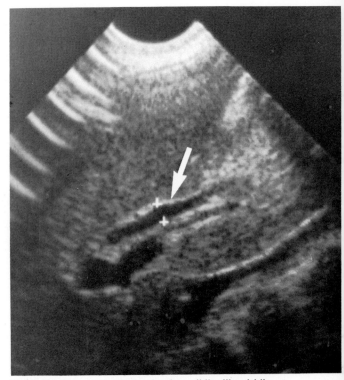

Fig. 5.18 Ultrasound of liver showing mildly dilated bile duct (→).

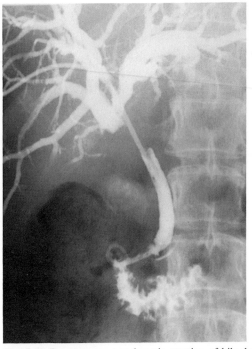

Fig. 5.19 Percutaneous transhepatic stenting of bile ducts to provide internal drainage in case of obstruction due to carcinoma of pancreas.

Table 5.1

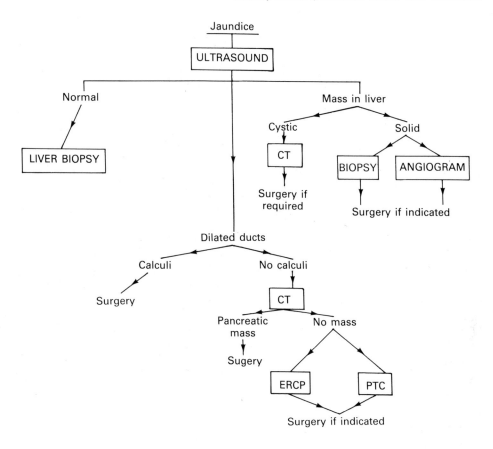

Pancreas

Only the exocrine aspects of the pancreas will be considered here, the endocrine diseases are dealt with in Chapter 8.

METHODS OF INVESTIGATION

Plain radiographs
The normal gland cannot be seen, but calcifications due to intraductal calculi or fat necrosis may be visible. Secondary effects of acute pancreatitis may also be demonstrated (q.v.)

Barium meal
The stomach or duodenum may be displaced or distorted by pancreatic swelling, masses or cysts.

Ultrasound
The head, body and much of the tail of the pancreas are visible on ultrasound (Figure 5.20). Intestinal gas may, however, obscure all or part of the gland, particularly if there is meteorism present. Ultrasound is especially useful in detecting and following cysts and pseudocysts.

Nuclear medicine
Concentration of selenomethionine in the pancreas indicates its exocrine activity, but being a non-specific test it has fallen into disuse.

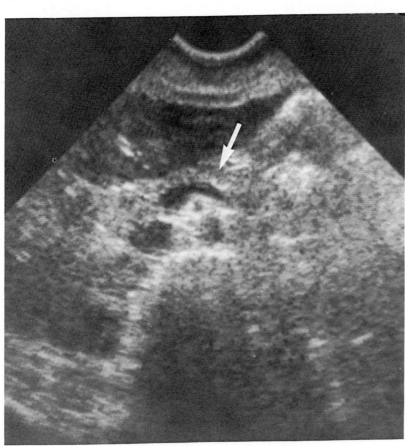

Fig. 5.20 Normal pancreas shown on transverse ultrasound of upper abdomen (→).

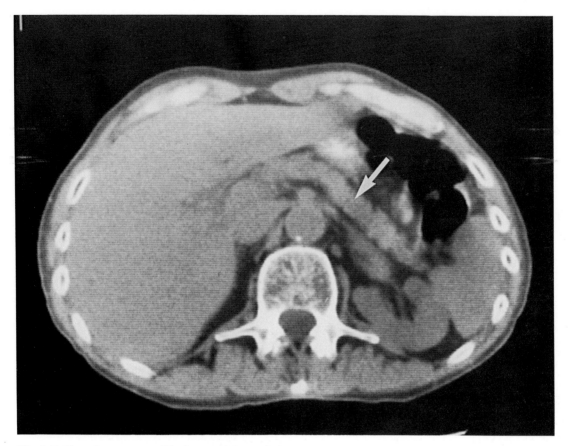

Fig. 5.21 Normal pancreas on CT of upper abdomen (→).

Computerized tomography
This technique always shows the pancreas and its adjacent structures well, and is the test of choice in most circumstances (Figure 5.21).

Endoscopic retrograde cholangio-pancreatography (ERCP)
An invasive procedure, ERCP permits cannulation via a gastroduodenoscope of the bile and pancreatic ducts, collection of duct fluid, and contrast ductography.

Angiography
Selective arteriography may demonstrate tumours, but with the other techniques available it is now rarely necessary.

LESIONS OF THE PANCREAS

ACUTE PANCREATITIS
In general, the diagnosis of acute pancreatitis is made clinically in the presence of raised serum amylase, but imaging is often required either to establish the diagnosis or to check for complications.

Radiological appearances
   1. Plain radiographs. Supine and erect films of the abdomen may show little in mild cases, but as the severity increases the following may be shown:
      (a) Loss of the psoas shadows.
      (b) Meteorism.

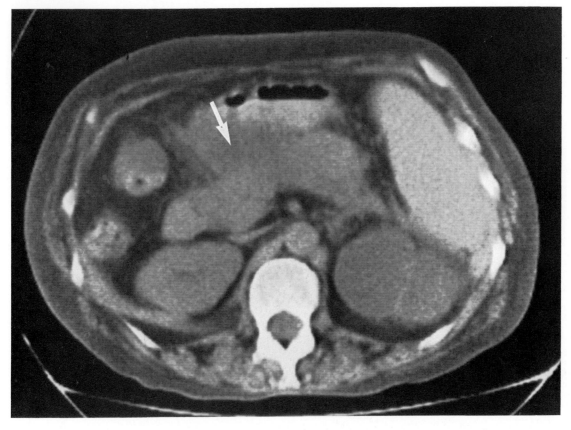

Fig. 5.22 Acute pancreatitis on CT. There is swelling of the gland and oedema of anterior tissues (→).

(c) The cut-off sign (absence of gas) in the transverse colon due to oedema of the transverse mesocolon.

(d) Dystrophic calcification in areas of fat necrosis.

(e) The presence of gallstones which are important in the aetiology.

(f) A chest film may show an elevated left hemidiaphragm, with left lower lobe consolidation and a small left pleural effusion.

2. Ultrasound: if the pancreas is visible through intestinal gas, it will be seen to be enlarged and oedematous. Sonolucencies in or adjacent to the gland may indicate cysts or pseudocysts which can be followed to check on their size, with or without drainage.

3. Computerized tomography: the gland is seen to be large and oedematous with adjacent tissue oedema and sometimes haemorrhage or fat necrosis (Figure 5.22). Cysts and pseudocysts are well seen.

4. Barium meal: swelling of the head of the gland will distort the duodenal loop. Pseudocysts in the lesser sac and structures near the stomach will also cause displacement and distortion of the stomach or duodenum.

CHRONIC PANCREATITIS

Differentiation between chronic pancreatitis and other chronic upper abdominal diseases is often difficult and may require many tests.

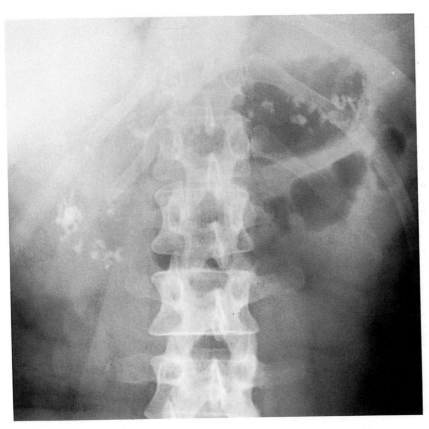

Fig. 5.23 Calculi in pancreas on plain radiograph in case of chronic pancreatitis.

Radiological appearances

1. Plain radiographs: the presence of pancreatic calculi (Figure 5.23) is pathognomonic of chronic pancreatitis, but occurs in only about 10% of cases.

2. Ultrasound: the pancreas is small, but the appearances are indistinguishable from atrophy unless calcification is present. The test is neither sensitive nor specific.

3. Computerized tomography: the changes are similar to those of ultrasound, but computerized tomography is more sensitive for calcification than either ultrasound or plain films (Figure 5.24)

4. *ERCP*: low volume secretion with poor enzyme concentration and the presence of irregular dilatation and strictures of the ducts may be found and are common in chronic pancreatitis (Fig. 5.25).

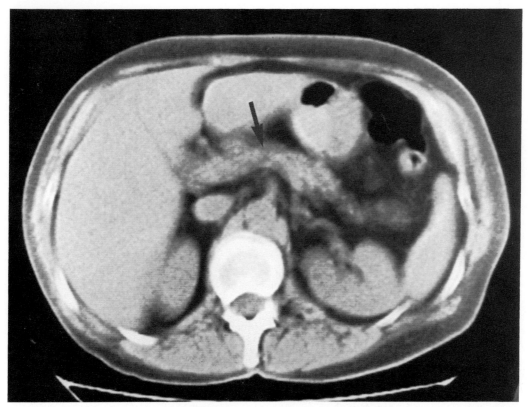

Fig. 5.24 Calcified chronic pancreatitis on CT (→).

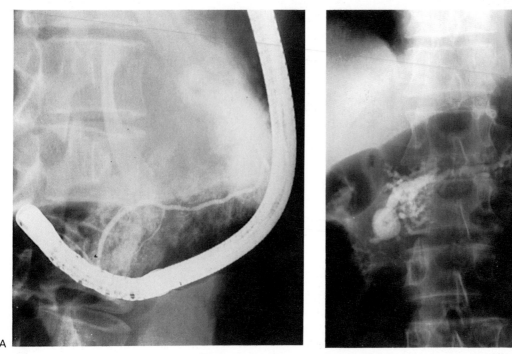

A

B

Fig. 5.25 (A) Normal pancreatic duct at ERCP. (B) Beaded pancreatic duct in chronic pancreatitis, demonstrated by ERCP.

ATROPHY

This is a relatively common process in old age, producing reduction in volume of the gland, but without calculi or duct distortion.

NEOPLASM

The most common neoplasm of the pancreas is adenocarcinoma of the exocrine glands. It usually presents with pain and/or jaundice.

Radiological appearances

1. Plain radiographs: these are generally normal. A chest film should be obtained to check for lung metastases.
2. Barium meal. A mass in the head of the pancreas may stretch the duodenal loop producing the 'reversed 3' sign, as described on page 106.
3. Ultrasound: a mass in the head or body of the gland in excess of 1 cm may be visible, but lesions in the tail are poorly seen.
4. Computerized tomography: the sensitivity is better than with ultrasound as the whole of the gland is visible. Extension of a tumour into the surrounding tissues or lymph nodes may be seen and is a bad prognostic sign (Figure 5.26).
5. Angiography: this is now rarely used except in cases with suspected tumours with hormonal excretion.
6. ERCP: This may show tumour cells in the duct secretions, and ductal distortion.

A suggested sequence of examinations for carcinoma of the pancreas is shown in Diagnostic decision tree 5, page 304.

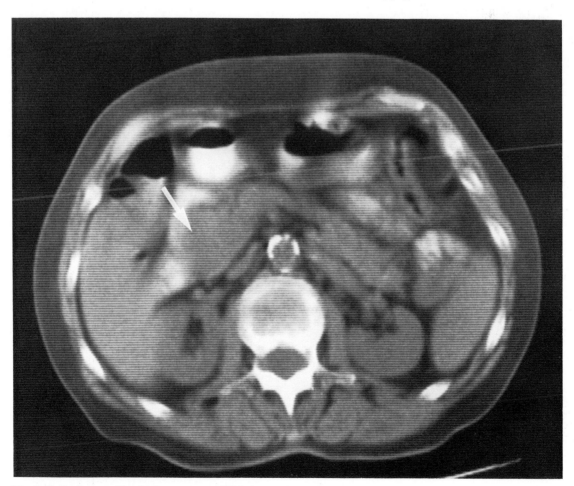

Fig. 5.26 Carcinoma of head of pancreas, on CT (→).

6 Skeletal System

METHODS OF INVESTIGATION

Plain radiographs
Plain radiographs are by far the most common method of demonstration of bones and joints.

Radionuclide scanning
Changes in local vascularity due to any pathological process are revealed by radionuclide scanning.

Tomography
An examination frequently used to show a lesion more clearly or to reveal changes which may be present within an area of sclerosis.

Angiography
Opacification of blood vessels may be used to investigate a suspected tumour.

Arthrography
The internal architecture of joints is demonstrated by arthrography. The cartilaginous and synovial surfaces of joints cannot be imaged directly except to a limited extent by computerized tomography and magnetic resonance imaging. More detailed study requires the injection of a water-soluble contrast medium, with or without additional gas which may be either air or carbon dioxide, to distend the joint and provide double contrast (Figure 6.1). All synovial joints, including shoulder, hip, ankle, wrist and interphalangeal joints, can be studied arthrographically, but the most commonly investigated joint is the knee. The indications are broad, but are usually related to meniscal damage of traumatic or, more rarely, of a degenerative nature. Osteochondritis and Baker's cysts, either intact or ruptured, are also clearly seen.

Computerized tomography
This is particularly useful in examinations of the skull, spine and pelvis.

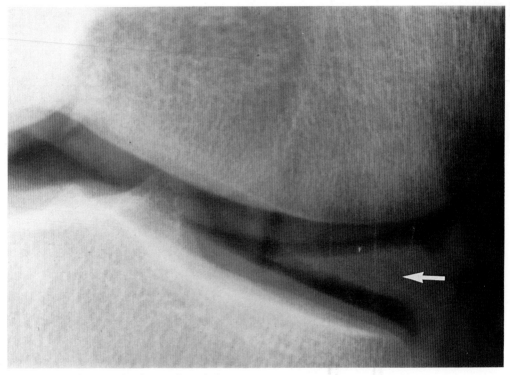

Fig. 6.1 Air arthrogram showing meniscus (→).

CONGENITAL ANOMALIES

There are a very large number of congenital anomalies of the skeleton but only those which are relatively common are dealt with here.

MADELUNG'S DEFORMITY
Due to failure of growth of the inner part of the distal radial epiphysis, the radius is short and bowed and the longer ulna projects posteriorly.

CONGENITAL DISLOCATION OF THE HIP
Usually unilateral, it is more common in females than males. Early recognition usually produces very good results of treatment. At that stage there is no ossification centre for the femoral capital epiphysis and lesser degrees of dislocation may not be recognized radiologically. Clinical examination with demonstration of the 'Ortolani' click is, however, usually reliable in diagnosis.

Radiological appearances (Figure 6.2)
Early:
    1. A shallow, vertical acetabulum.
Later:
    2. Upward and lateral displacement of the femoral head.
    3. Delayed ossification of the femoral capital epiphysis.
    4. Geometric assessments.

von Rosen's line
A radiograph is made of the baby's pelvis with the legs extended, internally rotated and abducted to 45°. A line drawn along the long axis of the femoral shaft and extended proximally will then pass through the lumbo-sacral joint in the normal child but lateral to this joint if there is fairly marked dislocation present. Geometric methods such as this, and estimating the angle made by the acetabulum with the horizontal, depend on precise positioning; in practice, an estimate of the

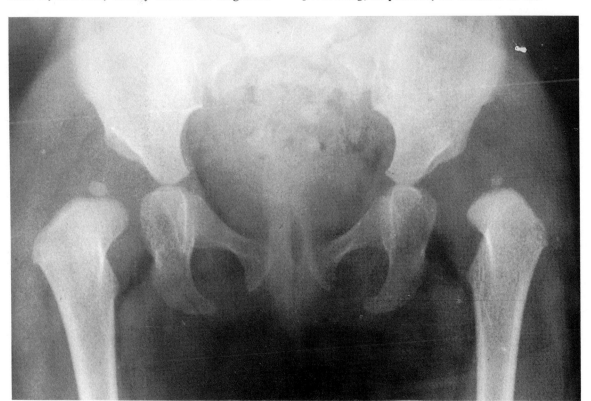

Fig. 6.2 Bilateral congenital hip dislocation showing lateral displacement of upper ends of femora, and dysplasia of acetabula.

position of the ossification centre of the femoral head in relation to the acetabulum on a radiograph of the child lying supine with both legs extended together and neither abducted nor adducted is often used.

MULTIPARTITE PATELLA
The patella is separated into two or more pieces. The condition is often bilateral which may assist in deciding whether the appearances of a patella are the result of a fracture or of a congenital anomaly. Unlike a fracture, the margins of the fragments are usually smooth and have a cortex.

HEMIVERTEBRA
Only the right or left half of a vertebra is present.

SPINA BIFIDA
There is failure of fusion of the two halves of the neural arch so that there is a gap in the arch at the spinous process (Figure 6.3). Minor forms are not important and may later fuse but gross gaps may be associated with a meningocele which projects through the gap. Neuropathic joints and hydrocephalus may be associated with gross cases.

SPONDYLOLISTHESIS
The *pars interarticularis* is the name given to the pillar of bone between the upper and lower articular facets on each side of a vertebra. In cases of spondylolisthesis there is a gap in the pars interarticularis on both sides of the vertebra. These gaps allow the anterior portion of the vertebra, comprising the body, pedicles and superior articular facets, to side forward away from the remainder of the vertebra (Figure 6.4). The gaps in the pars interarticularis are best seen in oblique views of the vertebra. The condition occurs most commonly at the lumbo-sacral junction and a lateral view of the area shows the body of L5 projecting forward in relation to the body of S1. There is often narrowing of the disc space between L5 and the sacrum. There appear to be two main causes for the gaps in the pars interarticularis:

1. A congenital failure of fusion of the upper and lower parts of the pars interarticularis

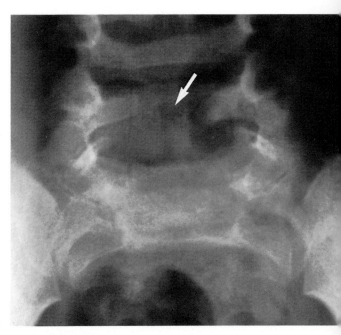

Fig. 6.3 Spina bifida at L5 (→).

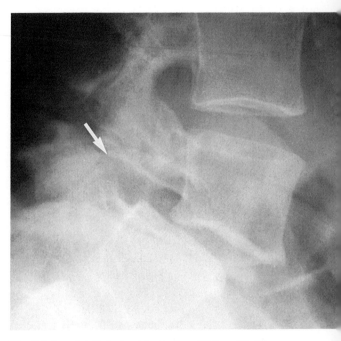

Fig. 6.4 Spondylolisthesis with slipping of L5 on S1. The pars interarticularis defect of L5 is shown (→).

2. Stress fractures of the pars interarticularis on each side of the vertebra.

The forward slip of the anterior segment of the vertebra results in narrowing of the neural formina with possible compression of the contained nerve roots. Occasionally gaps are present without displacement of the anterior segment of the vertebra and this condition is called *spondylolysis*.

RIB ANOMALIES
There may be additional ribs present or an absent rib. Additional ribs may be associated with hemivertebrae.

Cervical rib
This rib arises from the seventh cervical vertebra and may be large or rudimentary. The rudimentary rib may have a fibrous band between its free end and the first rib which may cause problems with the brachial plexus or the axillary artery.

SKELETAL DYSPLASIAS

OSTEOGENESIS IMPERFECTA (FRAGILITAS OSSIUM)
In this condition the bones are very fragile and fracture easily. It is the result of diminished osteoblastic activity. Fractures may be visible when the baby is still *in utero*. It may be associated with blue sclerotics, translucent and poorly developed teeth and prominent bulging of the skull in various regions.

Radiological appearances
1. Long bones show a thin cortex and little spongy bone (Figure 6.5). They tend to be more slender than normal. Deformities due to old fractures are common, but fractures when present heal by the normal processes.
2. The skull shows many Wormian bones along the suture lines.
3. The vertebrae are biconcave and less opaque than normal.

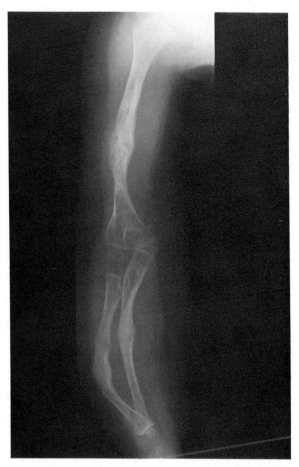

Fig. 6.5 Fragilitas ossium, with multiple healed fractures.

CLEIDOCRANIAL DYSOSTOSIS
A congenital condition which is characterized by defective formation of the clavicles and pubic bones and defective ossification of the skull.

Radiological appearances
1. Clavicles may be absent or present only in part. The outer end is most frequently missing.
2. Skull: the fontanelles and suture lines tend to remain open, and due to deficient ossification the sutures are wide.
3. Pubis: there may be deficient formation of the pubic bones, particularly in the region of the symphysis so that they are widely separated.
4. Spine: spina bifida is common.
5. Teeth: eruption of the teeth is delayed and the teeth may be poorly formed.

OSTEOPETROSIS

Calcified cartilage formed during the growth of
the bone fails to be absorbed and persists. The
bones are usually very brittle and transverse
fractures are common.

Radiological appearances

1. Thick bands of marked density are first
seen in the region of the metaphysis and these
bands later expand to involve the whole bone.

2. There is loss of definition of cortex and
medulla in the affected areas.

3. The vertebrae show dense zones in the
upper and lower part of the vertebral body and
these areas tend to expand and later involve the
whole of the vertebra.

4. Both the vault and base of the skull are
much more opaque than normal and the changes
in the base may cause narrowing of the
foramina.

DIAPHYSEAL ACLASIS (MULTIPLE EXOSTOSES)

This is usually an inherited and familial
condition which tends to become apparent in
late childhood.

Radiological appearances

1. Multiple exostoses with a well-defined
cortex around cancellous bone. The tip of the
exostosis has a cartilage cap which may calcify
and become very dense. The cartilage cap may
also undergo malignant change. In long bones
the exostoses occur at the metaphysis and point
away from the growing end of the bone. The
most common sites are around the knee and the
shoulder, but many other bones may be affected
(Figure 6.6).

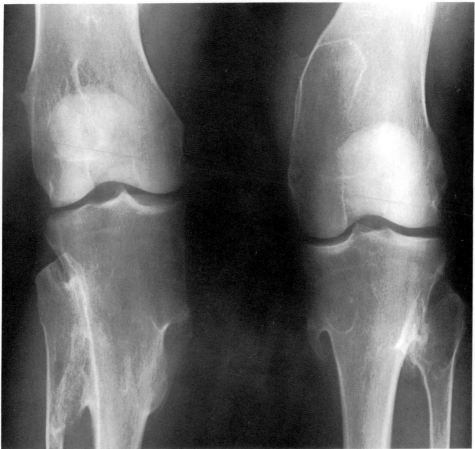

Fig. 6.6 Multiple exostoses around knee.

2. Irregular expansion of the long bone in the metaphyseal region.

3. The epiphyses are not affected in any way.

4. Deformity of the forearm. The ulna is short and pointed at the lower end. The radial head may be dislocated and the epiphysis at its lower end poorly formed.

ACHONDROPLASIA

This form of dwarfism results from retardation of endochondral ossification of bones formed from cartilage. Sub-periosteal bone formation is unaffected.

Radiological appearances

1. Limb bones: (a) short bones which are widened in the region of the metaphyses — bones of the hands and feet are involved as well as the long bones; (b) muscular attachments are enlarged.

2. Skull: (a) the vault is normal; (b) the base is unusually short; (c) the mandible is of normal size and so juts forwards.

3. Spine: (a) the vertebrae are normal or slightly wedged; (b) there is usually a lordosis of the lumbar spine.

4. Pelvis: the inlet is contracted and the internal measurements diminished.

FIBROUS DYSPLASIA

In this condition areas of bone are replaced by fibrous tissue. It may affect single or multiple bones. It may be associated with precocious puberty, particularly in females, and with accompanying skin pigmentation — Albright's syndrome. Fibrous dysplasia commences in childhood but is often not recognized until later in life when a pathological fracture occurs.

Radiological appearances

1. Well-defined cyst-like areas which have a ground glass appearances (Figure 6.7).

2. Expansion of bone — particularly flat bones.

3. Epiphyses are not affected until after they have fused.

4. In the skull the facial bones and base may be affected and become very sclerotic.

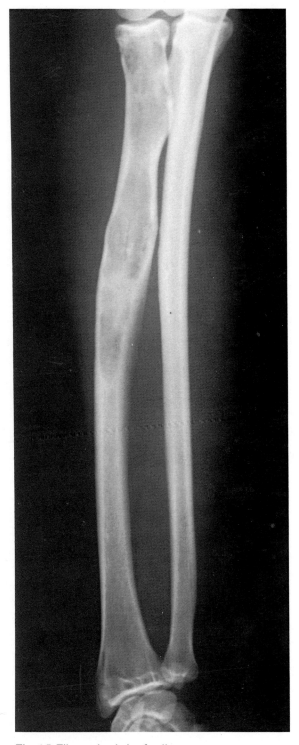

Fig. 6.7 Fibrous dysplasia of radius.

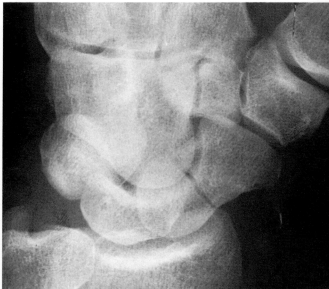

Fig. 6.8 Fracture of waist of carpal scaphoid.

TRAUMATIC LESIONS

Only relatively common traumatic conditions are dealt with in this chapter.

Some undisplaced fractures, such as occur in the carpal scaphoid, may not be apparent immediately after injury and only become obvious after 10–14 days when resorption of bone along the fracture surfaces occurs (Figure 6.8). In the vast majority of cases of fractures of the extremities two views of the fracture at right angles, usually an antero-posterior and a lateral view, are the minimal requirement. Oblique views may also be necesary.

In children fractures of long bones may be of the 'greenstick' type in which the fracture is incomplete and the bone simply appears to be bent at the site of the injury (Figure 6.9).

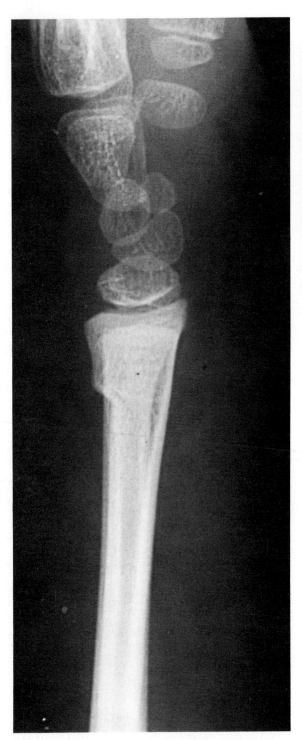

Fig. 6.9 Greenstick Colles' fracture of radius. Lateral projection.

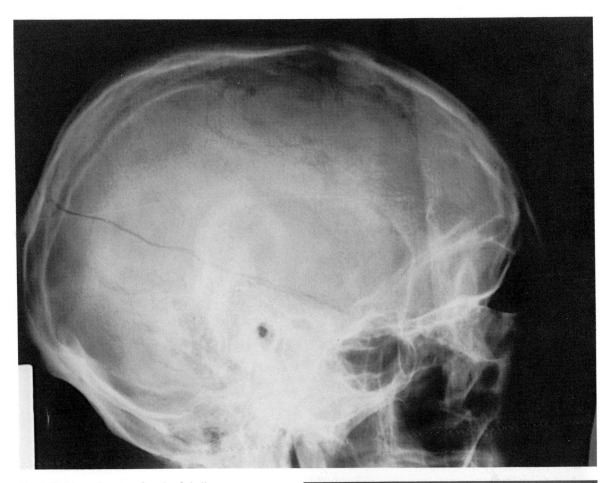

Fig. 6.10 Linear fracture of vault of skull.

THE SKULL

Linear fractures

Radiological appearances (Figure 6.10)

1. Linear dark shadows — darker than vascular or sutural markings.

2. The fracture lines do not branch.

3. The factures often run in a direction not usual for vascular markings.

Depressed fractures

Radiological appearances (Figure 6.11)

1. They appear as dense white lines due to overlap of bone.

2. Tangential views show the depressed bone.

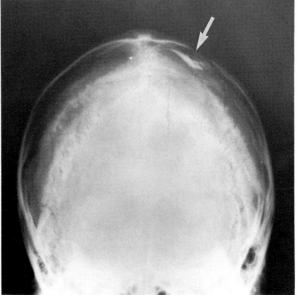

Fig. 6.11 Depressed fracture of skull (→).

Facial fractures

For the purposes of description the face can be divided into three areas, a central third and two lateral thirds.

Lateral fractures

1. Slight injury to the lateral side of the face may result in fracture and depression of the zygomatic arch.

2. A more severe blow will push the malar bone into the antrum. The antrum appears small by comparison with the antrum on the other side and fractures are visible in the floor of the orbit and in the lateral wall of the antrum. The frontozygomatic suture is opened up (Figure 6.12).

Central fractures

René Le Fort classified major fractures into three main types (Figure 6.13):

1. Le Fort I fracture. A transverse fracture through the maxilla just above the teeth.

2. Le Fort II fracture. A pyramidal fracture frees the whole of the central block of facial bones from its attachments. The fracture lines commence at the frontonasal suture and run downwards and laterally, often through the inferior orbital foramen and through the anterior and lateral walls of the antrum. The whole block of freed bone may be depressed.

3. Le Fort III fracture. A high transverse fracture may occur with the fracture line passing across the face at the level of the nasal bones and separating the facial bones from the base of the skull.

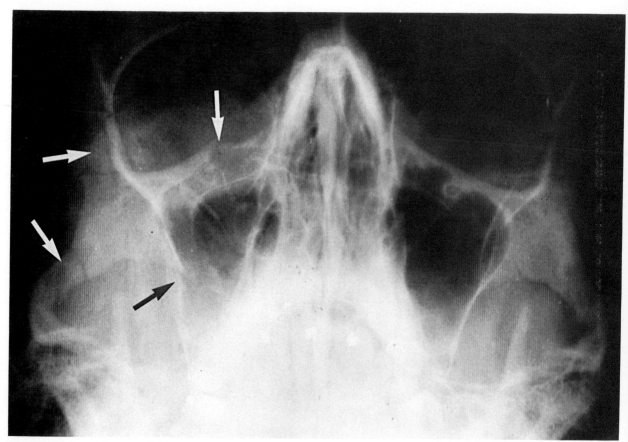

Fig. 6.12 Depressed fracture of right malar.
There are fractures of the inferior orbital margin, lateral wall of maxillary antrum, and zygomatic arch, and diastasis of the fronto-malar synchondrosis (→).

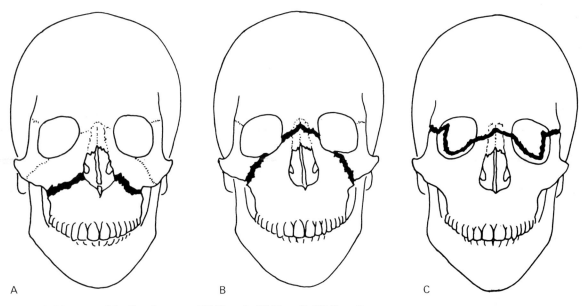

Fig. 6.13 Diagrams of Le Fort fractures. (A) Type 1; (B) Type 2; (C) Type 3.

Blow-out fractures

A direct blow to the orbit may result in a fracture of the floor and/or medial wall of the orbit. Orbital contents may escape through the floor and be visible as an area of opacity in the upper part of the antrum (Figure 6.14) or through the medial wall when the ethmoid cells will become opaque. These fractures are often best shown by computerized tomography scanning but may be visible on plain films or tomograms.

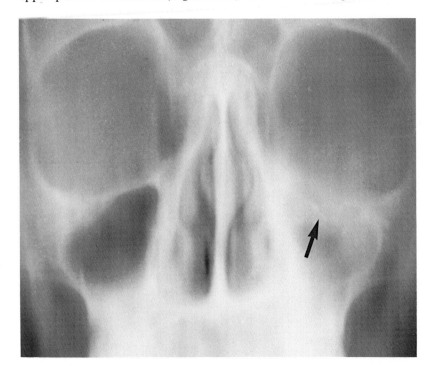

Fig. 6.14 Tomograph of blowout fracture of floor of left orbit (→).

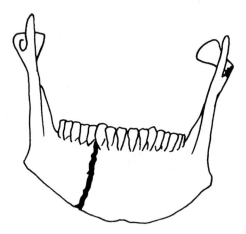

Fig. 6.15 Diagram of fracture of mandible.

Nasal bone fractures
These are best seen in soft tissue lateral and supero-inferior views, which also show the degree of displacement.

Mandibular fractures
The common sites of fracture are through the region of the canine tooth and through the neck of the bone. It is common for both of these fractures to occur together and they may be present on opposite sides of the mandible (Figure 6.15).

THE SPINE
The common spinal fracture, particularly in the dorsal and lumbar areas, is anterior wedging of a vertebral body, but different regions of the spine have specific fractures and dislocations, all of which may cause damage to the spinal cord.

Cervical spine
1. Fracture of the odontoid process. The fracture usually occurs through the base of the process and the odontoid and atlas may be dislocated forwards or backwards (Figure 6.16a).
2. Rupture of the transverse ligament of the atlas. This allows the second cervical vertebra to move backwards (Figure 6.16b).
3. Fracture of the neural arch of the second cervical vertebra (Figure 6.16c). This allows forward dislocation of this vertebra on C3.

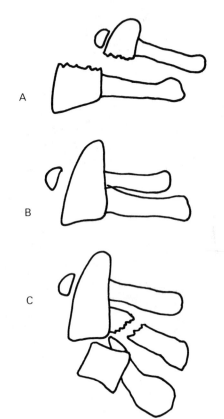

Fig. 6.16 Diagrams of fractures of upper cervical spine.
(A) Fractured odontoid process.
(B) Ruptured transverse ligament with posterior displacement of C2.
(C) Fractured arch of C2, with displacement of the body of C2 relative to C3.

4. Whip-lash injuries. These may result in fractures of cervical spinous processes, or in narrowing of cervical discs, or may show no radiological abnormality.

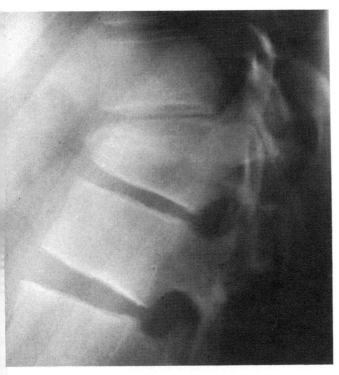

Fig. 6.17 Old wedge fracture of thoracic vertebra.

Thoracic spine

The common fracture of the thoracic spine is anterior wedging of vertebrae (Figure 6.17) often with narrowing of the adjacent intervertebral discs. This disc narrowing may not become apparent until months after the original injury.

Lumbar spine

It is common for the transverse processes to be fractured. Wedging of vertebral bodies and narrowing of adjacent discs may also occur. As in the thoracic spine, the narrowing may be delayed.

Disc narrowing

Narrowing of intervertebral discs is a common finding, particularly in the lumbar and cervical areas, and results most frequently from disc degeneration which may on occasion be the result of old trauma (Figure 6.18). The nucleus pulposus may herniate posteriorly and project into the spinal canal. In the early stages following

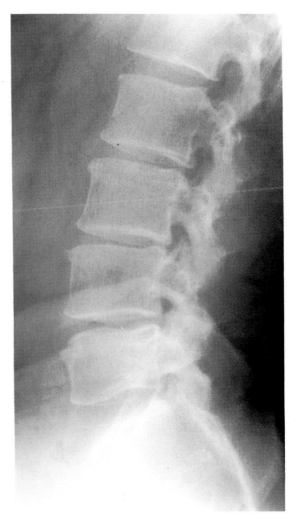

Fig. 6.18 Narrowing of lumbar intervertebral disc space due to degeneration.

trauma there is often no change on plain films but later there may be disc narrowing. The herniated nucleus is well shown by myelography, discography in which opaque material is injected into the disc space or by magnetic resonance imaging (Figure 6.19).

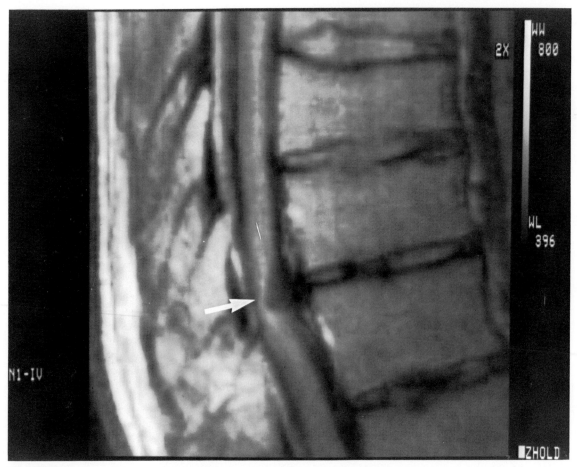

Fig. 6.19 Magnetic resonance image of thoracic spine showing disc protrusion (→).
(Philips Gyroscan, by courtesy of Philips Medical Systems Div, Eindhoven, The Netherlands).

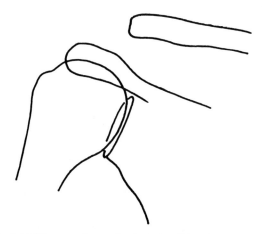

Fig. 6.20 Diagram of acromio-clavicular dislocation.

THE UPPER LIMB

The clavicle

Fractures
Fractures of the clavicle often have overlap of the fragments.

Subluxation
The sterno-clavicular joint is rarely dislocated but when this is present the clavicle is seen to be riding high at the joint by comparison with the position of the clavicle at the opposite joint. The joint space is wide due to upward displacement of the clavicle. Dislocation of the outer end of the clavicle upwards away from the acromion may occur (Figure 6.20).

The shoulder joint

Fractures
The most common fracture is through the surgical neck of the humerus but detachment of the greater tuberosity may also be seen. In children there may be separation of the capital epiphysis from the shaft (Figure 6.21).

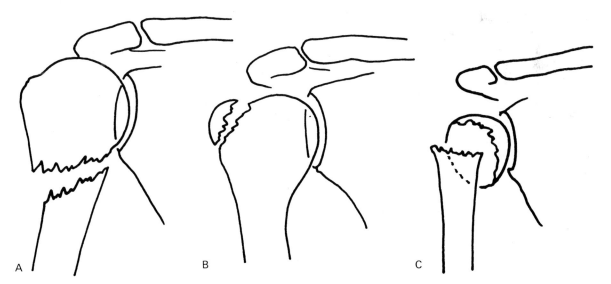

A   B   C

Fig. 6.21 Diagram of types of fractures of upper humerus:
(A) surgical neck; (B) greater tuberosity; (C) subcapital, with displacement.

Dislocations

Dislocations commonly result in the humeral head lying in front of the neck of the scapula or below the glenoid. Rarely the humeral head is displaced posteriorly and it then has a more rounded appearance in the antero-posterior view, and the joint space between the humerus and glenoid is lost. With recurrent dislocation of the shoulder joint a smooth depression often develops on the postero-lateral aspect of the humeral head (Figure 6.22).

Calcification

Chronic trauma may result in calcification in the supraspinatus tendon.

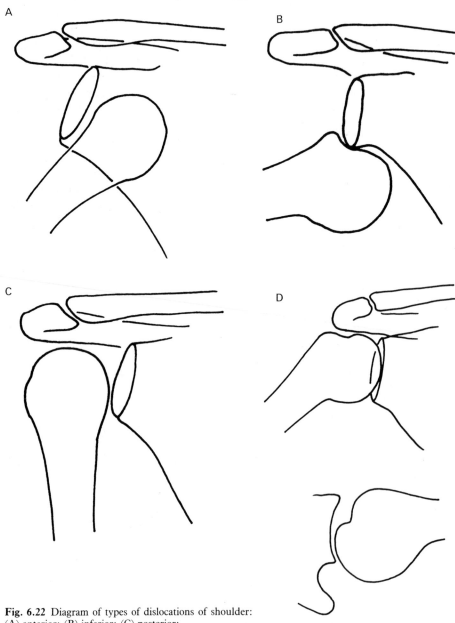

Fig. 6.22 Diagram of types of dislocations of shoulder:
(A) anterior; (B) inferior; (C) posterior;
(D) showing the notch due to recurrent dislocation.

The elbow joint

Fractures

The elbow joint is a common site for fractures in children.

1. Supracondylar (Figure 6.23a): in children, this is usually a transverse fracture immediately above the condyles of the humerus. In adults, it is usually a T-shaped fracture with the vertical limb passing down to the articular surface.

2. Medial epicondyle (Figure 6.23b): it is common in children for the medial epicondyle of the humerus to be avulsed and the detached fragment may be displaced into the elbow joint.

3. Distal humeral epiphysis (Figure 6.23c): the whole epiphysis may be loosened and slide forwards.

4. Head of radius (Figure 6.23d): vertical fractures occur through the head of the bone with often a downward displacement of a fragment creating a step in the articular surface.

5. Neck of radius (Figure 6.23d): the fracture is usually transverse and impaction of the fragments is common.

6. Head of ulna (Figure 6.23e): fractures are usually transverse through the olecranon process with often wide separation of the fragments.

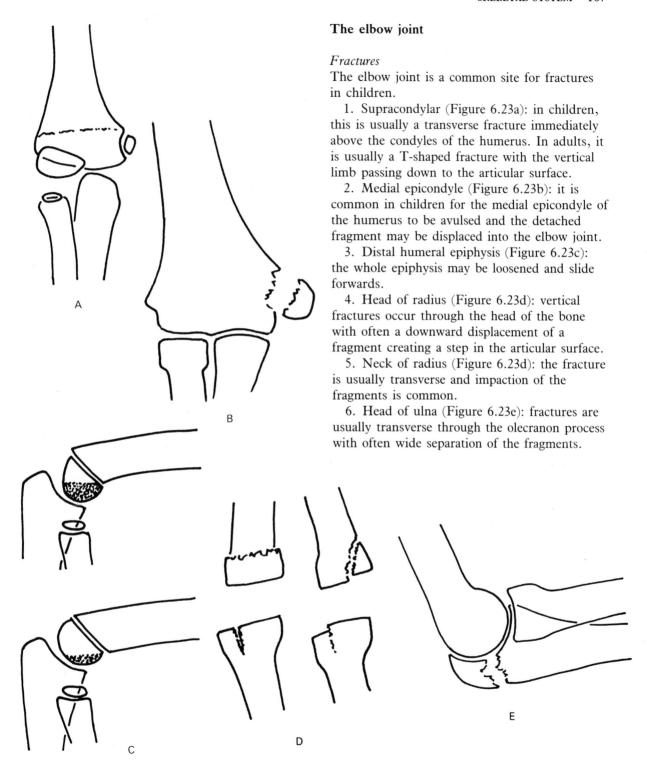

Fig. 6.23 Diagram of types of fractures of the elbow:
(A) supracondylar; (B) medial epicondylar; (C) displaced lower humeral epiphysis (normal for comparison);
(D) head of radius (several types); (E) olecranon process.

Dislocation

Commonly the radius and ulna are dislocated posteriorly and proximally to lie behind the humerus. A fracture of the coronoid process may accompany this dislocation (Figure 6.24).

The wrist joint

Fractures

1. Colles' fracture (Figure 6.25): a transverse fracture through the distal end of the radius with dorsal tilt of the distal fragment. Impaction of the fragments is common and the ulnar styloid is often detached.

2. Smith's fracture (reversed Colles'): this fracture is similar to a Colles' fracture but with forward rotation of the distal fragment.

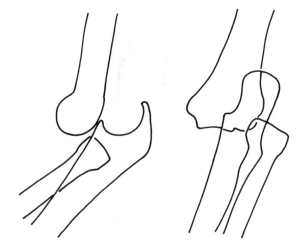

Fig. 6.24 Diagram of dislocation of elbow, lateral and AP views.

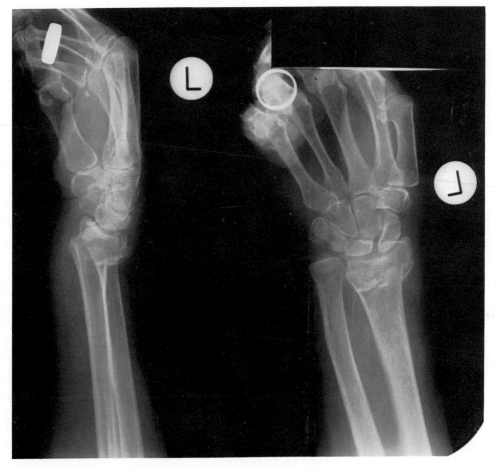

Fig. 6.25 Colles' fracture of wrist.

The carpus

Fractures

1. Scaphoid fractures usually occur through the waist of the bone (see Figure 6.8). There is often no significant displacement of the fragments and the fracture line may not become visible for 10–14 days when resorption of bone along the fracture line has occured. The fracture may interfere with the blood supply of the bone resulting in avascular necrosis of one fragment which then appears dense by comparison with the other fragment (Figure 6.26).

2. Triquetrum: detachment of flakes of bone from the dorsal aspect of this bone by ligamentous tearing is common.

Dislocations

Complex dislocations of the carpal bones may occur, but the common simple dislocation involves the lunate which rotates forwards so that the concave articular surface for the capitate now faces forwards. In the postero-anterior view the lunate assumes a triangular shape rather than its normal oblong form.

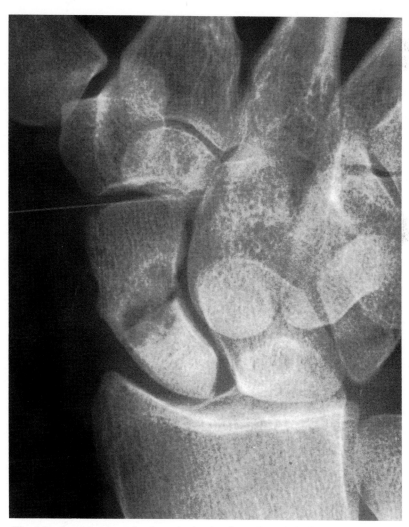

Fig. 6.26 Avascular necrosis of proximal pole of carpal scaphoid following trauma.

The hand

Bennett's fracture

A vertical fracture occurs through the anterior portion of the base of the first metacarpal which frees a fragment anteriorly and may allow the remainder of the bone to become dislocated posteriorly and proximally in relation to the trapezium (Figure 6.27).

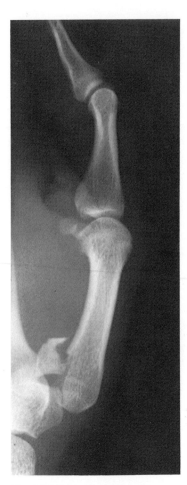

Fig. 6.27 Bennett's fracture of base of first metacarpal.

THE LOWER LIMB

The hip joint

Fractures

1. Abduction fracture (Figure 6.28a): the fracture line passes across the neck of the femur and the shaft of the bone is abducted in relation to the upper fragment. There is often impaction of the fragments.

2. Intertrochanteric fracture (Figure 6.28b): the fracture line runs between the femoral trochanters and the shaft is adducted in relation to the upper fragment. The lesser trochanter is often completely detached.

3. Subcapital fracture (Figure 6.28c): the fracture occurs at the junction of the head and neck of the femur. The shaft is often adducted and the fragments impacted.

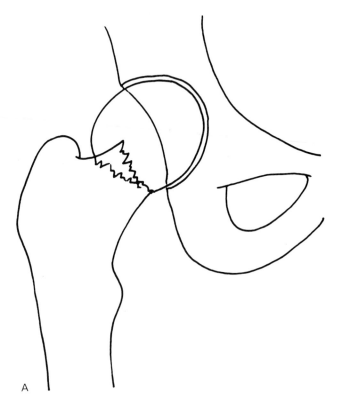

A

Fig. 6.28 Diagram of types of fractures of hip:
(A) abduction fracture of femoral neck;
(opposite page) (B) pertrochanteric fracture (adduction);
(C) subcapital.

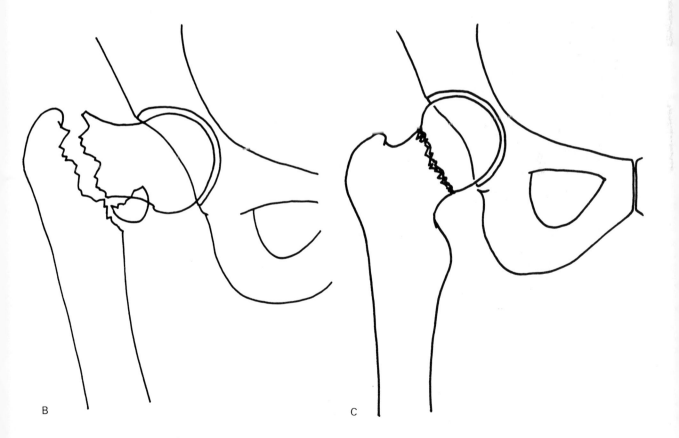

B

C

Dislocations

1. Posterior dislocation (Figure 6.29a): the head of the femur lies above and behind the acetabulum and an accompanying fracture of the posterior rim of the acetabulum is common.

2. Anterior dislocation (Figure 6.29b): the head of the femur lies anterior to and below the acetabulum.

3. Central dislocation (Figure 6.29c): a fracture through the upper part of the acetabulum allows the head of the femur to be displaced medially towards the pelvic cavity.

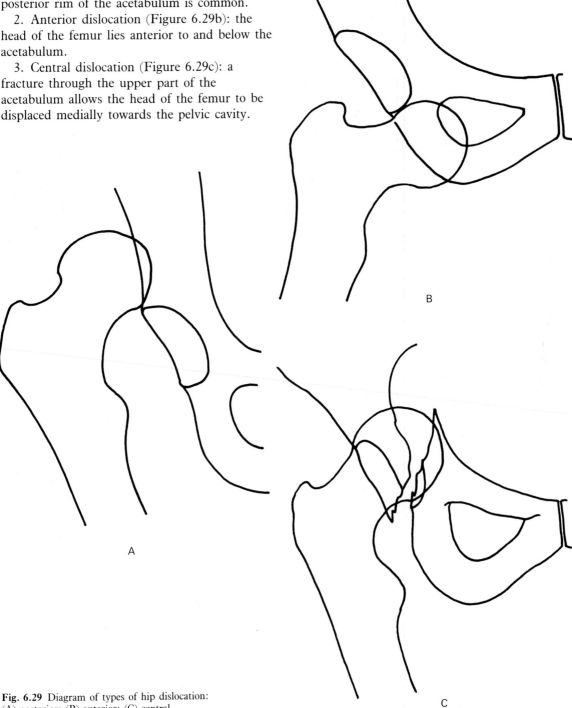

Fig. 6.29 Diagram of types of hip dislocation: (A) posterior; (B) anterior; (C) central.

Slipped femoral epiphysis

This condition, which is generally thought to result from repeated low grade trauma to the hip joint, tends to occur between the ages of 9 and 17 and to be more common in males than females. The patient usually presents with a painful limp of some months' standing, but which may have recently become worse.

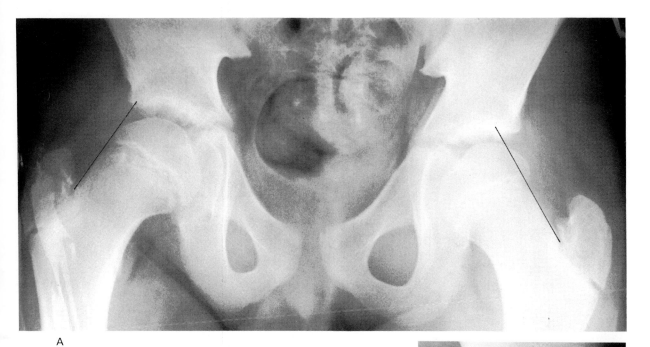

A

Radiological appearances (Figure 6.30)

1. The epiphysis for the head of the femur is displaced posteriorly and/or medially.

2. There is a band of translucency in the femoral neck distal to the epiphyseal line.

A line drawn along the upper margin of the neck of the femur in the antero-posterior projection passes through the edge of the capital epiphysis in the normal hip but passes lateral to the epiphysis when there is medial slip. In the lateral view the posterior displacement is visible.

Fig. 6.30 (A) Slipped right upper femoral epiphysis (left normal). (B) Lateral projection.

B

The pelvis

Fractures

The common fractures are through the superior and inferior pubic rami; these may be associated with a fracture in the region of the opposite sacro-iliac joint, or an opening up of that joint (Figure 6.31).

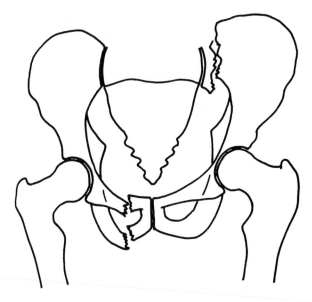

Fig. 6.31 Diagram of fractures of pelvis.

The knee joint

Fractures

1. Supracondylar femoral fracture (Figure 6.32a): the fracture occurs across the distal portion of the femoral shaft and often has a vertical limb running down to the femoral articular surface.

2. Lateral tibial condyle fracture (Figure 6.32b): the fracture line runs obliquely downwards and laterally from the tibial articular surface and isolates the lateral tibial condyle. This may be associated with a fracture of the neck of the fibula.

3. Patellar fracture: commonly the fracture line runs transversely across the patella and there is often wide separation of the fragments (Figure 6.32c). Rarely the fracture is star-shaped with several free fragments. It is important not to confuse a congenital bipartite or multipartite patella with a fracture. The margins of the fragments of a multipartite patella are smooth and have a well-defined cortex in contrast to the slightly irregular uncorticated margins of a fracture. The congenital anomaly is usually bilateral, which may help in cases of doubt.

4. Tibial spine: the spine of the tibia may be avulsed by stress on the cruciate ligaments (Figure 6.32d).

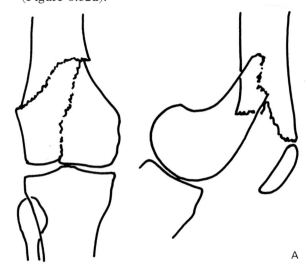

A

Fig. 6.32 Diagram of fractures of knee:
(A) supracondylar;
(opposite page) (B) lateral tibial plateau;
(C) patella;
(D) tibial spine.

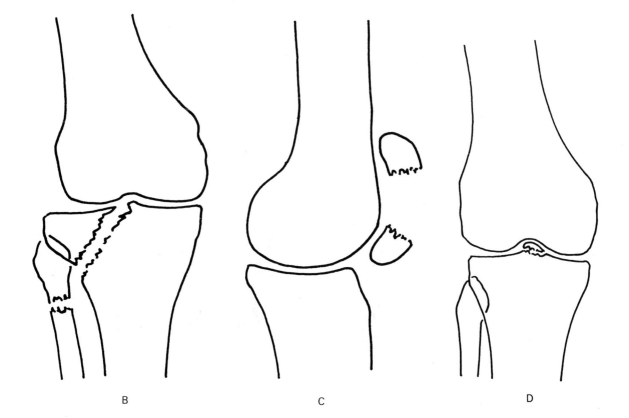

B   C   D

The ankle

Fractures

1. Pott's fracture — abduction type:
    (a) First degree. A fracture at the junction of shaft and lateral condyle of the fibula (Figure 6.33a).
    (b) Second degree. Fractures of both the lateral and medial malleoli with lateral displacement of the talus (Figure 6.33b).

    (c) Third degree. Fractures of the lateral and medial malleoli, a vertical fracture through the posterior tibial malleolus and posterior displacement of the talus (Figure 6.33c).

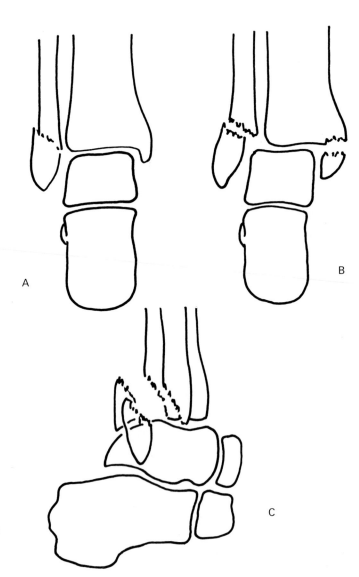

Fig. 6.33 Diagram of abduction fractures of ankle: (A) first degree; (B) second degree; (C) third degree.

2. Pott's fracture — adduction type:
   (a) First degree. An oblique fracture of the medial malleolus (Figure 6.34a).
   (b) Second degree. Fractures of the lateral and medial malleoli and medial displacement of the talus (Figure 6.34b).
   (c) Third degree. A fracture of the lateral and medial malleoli, a vertical fracture of the posterior tibial malleolus, and posterior displacement of the talus (Figure 6.34c).

Ligamentous damage
Rupture of the lateral ligament of the ankle joint will lead to an unstable joint. The diagnosis is made by making an antero-posterior view of the joint during forced inversion of the foot when the talus will be seen to rotate inside the mortice of the ankle joint.

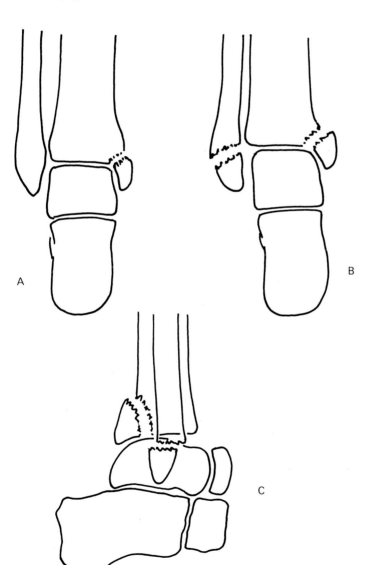

A

B

C

Fig. 6.34 Diagram of adduction fractures of ankle: (A) first degree; (B) second degree; (C) third degree.

The foot

Fractures

1. Calcaneal fractures: the angle between a line drawn across the margins of the upper surface of the calcaneus and a line drawn across the margins of the articular surface for the talus should be not more than 140°. An increase in this angle suggests the presence of a fracture (Figure 6.35). A crush fracture of the calcaneus may also cause splaying of the bone when viewed from above.

2. Talus fractures: fracture may occur through the neck of the bone with either slight or marked separation of the fragments and with a small fragment often detached from the anterior aspect of the tibial articular surface (Figure 6.36).

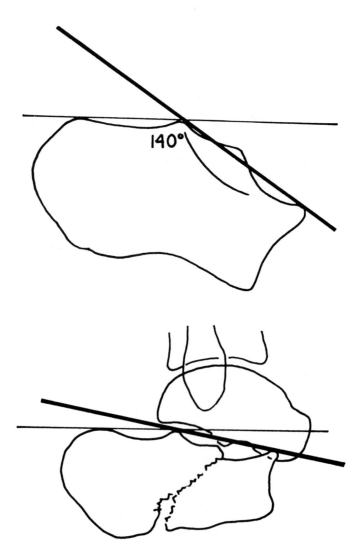

Fig. 6.35 Diagram of fracture of os calcis, with normal for comparison, showing flattening of Bohler's angle.

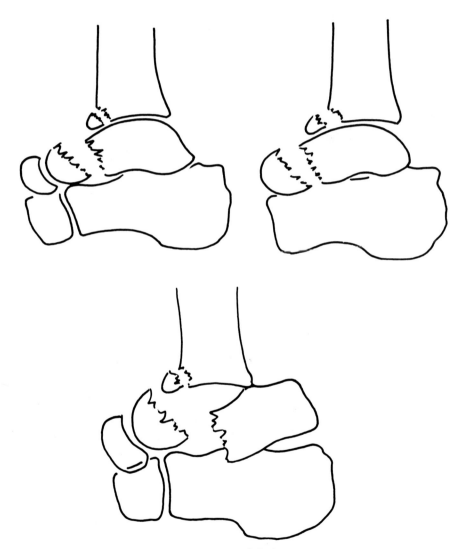

Fig. 6.36 Diagram of fractures of the talus, of varying degrees of displacement.

BONE LESIONS OF UNKNOWN AETIOLOGY

OSTEOCHONDRITIS

Epiphyseal osteochondritis is generally regarded as being due to an avascular necrosis although the causes of the avascularity are not clear. It has been suggested that it results from chronic trauma. Many epiphyses can be affected and sometimes more than one can be involved in the same patient. The common types only will be discussed.

Femoral capital epiphysis (Perthes–Legg–Calvé's disease)

The condition usually occurs between 3 and 14 years with a maximum incidence between 6 and 8 years and is more common in males than females; the patient usually presents with a painful limp. A feature of the condition is that the radiological findings are often much worse than the clinical state would suggest, but the reverse may also be true. As well as arising *de novo* it may accompany many other diseases, the most notable of which is probably congenital dislocation of the hip.

Radiological appearances
Early:
   1. Slightly increased density of the epiphysis.
   2. Osteoporosis of the neighbouring part of the femur.
   3. Widening of the hip joint space due to cartilage proliferation.
Later:
   4. The epiphysis becomes fragmented and flattened (Figure 6.37).
   5. A band of translucency in the metaphysis.
   6. The neck of the femur becomes widened.

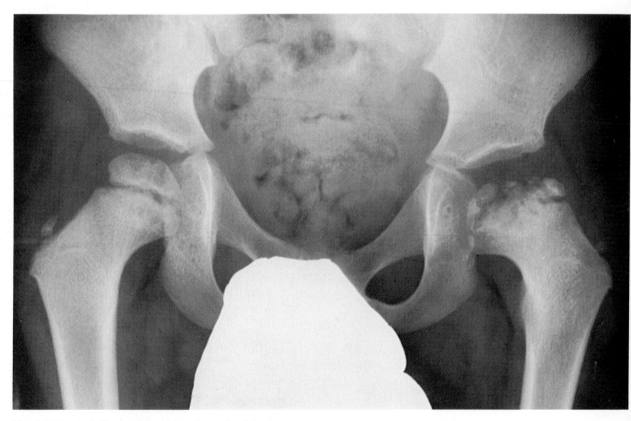

Fig. 6.37 Perthes' disease of the hip, early on the right, but severe with fragmentation of the epiphysis on the left.

With healing, which occupies 2–3 years, the normal shape and bone pattern of the epiphysis are restored in some cases, but in the majority there is usually some widening of the femoral neck and enlargement of the femoral head which in later years may lead to osteoarthritic changes in the hip.

Tarsal navicular
Fragmentation and increased density develop and the bone undergoes compression in the antero-posterior diameter, which may be extremely marked. With healing, the size, shape, and texture of the bone become completely re-established.

Metatarsal head
The second metatarsal is usually affected and the changes may occur before or after fusion of the epiphysis. The head of the bone becomes dense and fragmented and the adjacent surfaces of the metatarsal and proximal phalanx become expanded. New bone forms along the metatarsal shaft.

OSTEOCHONDRITIS DISSECANS
This occurs chiefly in young adults, but may occur in later years and is the most common cause of a loose body in the joints of young people. It affects many sites such as the knee, elbow and ankle, but is most common at the medial condyle of the femur.

Radiological appearances (Figure 6.38)

1. A circular radiolucent area appears around a fragment of bone on the articular surface and when seen in profile, the fragment is seen to lie in a small depression in the bone.

2. The fragment of bone with its overlying articular cartilage may become free within the joint or it may remain *in situ* and later become absorbed.

3. Sometimes only the cartilage is involved and a loose body so formed needs arthrography to demonstrate its presence.

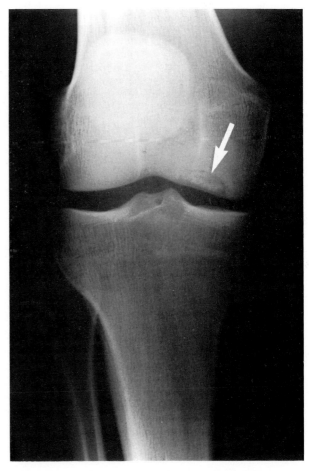

Fig. 6.38 Osteochondritis diseccans of the medial femoral condyle (→).

PAGET'S DISEASE

This is a disease of unknown origin, affecting bones in the middle and late age groups and which is more common in men than in women. The bones most commonly affected are the pelvis, lumbar spine, femur and tibia. The hands and feet are rarely affected. Radiologically there are two types: amorphous and spongy.

Radiological appearances (Figure 6.39)

1. The amorphous type shows a loss of normal bone pattern and a uniform grey appearance of the bones.

2. The spongy type also shows a loss of normal bone pattern which is replaced by an irregular coarse trabeculation.

Both types show the following changes:

3. Enlargement of bones due to marked cortical thickening.

4. A V-shaped junction of normal and abnormal areas in long bones.

5. The bones are soft, resulting in bowing of the femur and tibia and deformity of the pelvis due to inward protrusion of the acetabuli — protrusio acetabuli.

6. Pseudo-fractures may be present on the convex surface of bowed long bones. These are breaks in the continuity of the bone which extend for varying distances into the shaft and which have sclerotic margins.

7. Skull changes. Two types of change occur in the vault: (a) areas of increased density in the outer table with marked thickening of the bones and loss of the definition between the two tables (Figure 6.40); (b) a large irregular area of osteoporosis, usually in the frontal region — osteoporosis circumscripta (Figure 6.41).

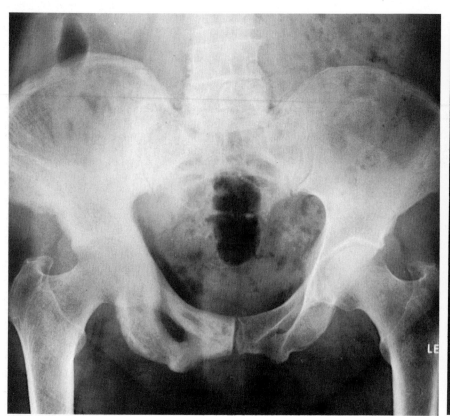
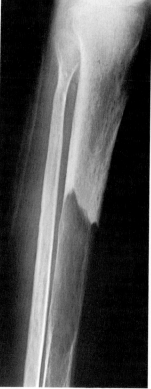

Fig. 6.39 (A) Sclerotic Paget's disease of right side of pelvis. (B) Amorphous Paget's disease of tibia, with typical 'flame-shaped' junction with normal bone.

A

B

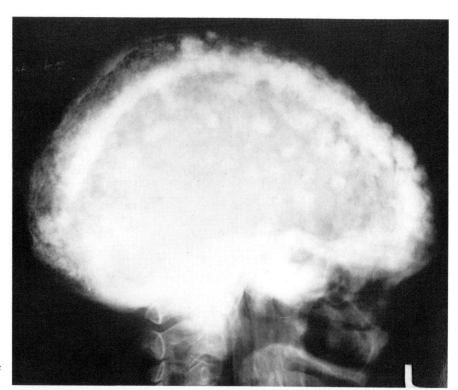

Fig. 6.40 Sclerotic Paget's disease of skull.

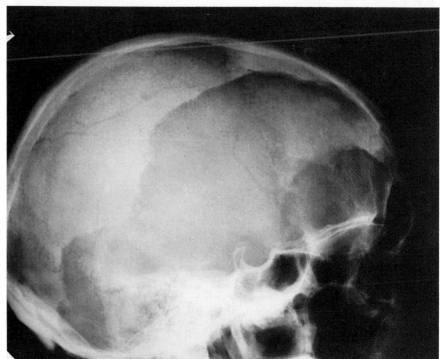

Fig. 6.41 Osteoporosis circumscripta. Amorphous Paget's disease of skull.

Complications
  1. Fracture: typical transverse fractures occur easily in long bones.
  2. Cranial nerve palsies: thickening and softening of the bones of the skull base may cause narrowing of the basal foramina, which may affect the contained nerves. The base of the skull may bulge up into the cranial cavity (basilar invagination).
  3. Sarcomatous changes, although uncommon, may develop in affected bones.
  4. High output cardiac failure may occur because of the very high degree of vascularity of the bones.

Differential diagnosis
Metastases in the skeletal pelvis and lumbar spine from a carcinoma of the prostate, and lymphomatous deposits in lumbar vertebrae may simulate Paget's disease. The serum acid phosphatase, however, is elevated with prostatic metastases.

INFANTILE CORTICAL HYPEROSTOSIS (CAFFEY'S DISEASE)
The disease is characterized by painful soft tissue swellings and bony thickening. It occurs before the age of 5 months and has been described *in utero*. The bones most commonly affected are the mandible, clavicle and scapula, but any bone may be involved except the phalanges.

Radiological appearances
There is marked cortical thickening of bone underlying the soft tissue masses. The appearances return to normal within a year.

Differential diagnosis
Hypervitaminosis A produces similar changes but does not appear before 5 months.

BONE AND JOINT INFECTIONS

PERIOSTEAL REACTION
Apart from inflammatory change there are a large variety of conditions which cause elevation or thickening of the periosteum, and the reader is referred to other texts for a full account of these conditions.

The common causes are inflammation and trauma, but it also occurs with both primary and occasionally secondary neoplasms. The appearances in neoplasia are discussed under 'Bone tumours', page 202.

Periostitis
In coccal inflammatory diseases of bone, the earliest sign is usually elevation of the periosteum in the area affected. This elevated periosteum appears as a fine white line running parallel to and separated from the bone by a thin black line due to the inflammatory exudate which is lifting the periosteum off the bone.

OSTEOMYELITIS
This is most commonly caused by haematogenous spread, usually of a staphylococcus, from a skin infection. Other blood-bone infective agents such as streptococci are occasionally responsible, or there may be spread to the bone from a neighbouring soft tissue or joint infection.

Acute osteomyelitis

Radiological appearances (Figure 6.42)
  1. No change is apparent for 10–14 days after the onset of symptoms.
  2. Elevation of the periosteum over a section of the bone is the early sign.
  3. Sometimes there may be seen an ill-defined area of oesteoporosis underlying the raised periosteum.
  4. Obliteration of the soft tissue planes in the area due to oedema.
  Radionuclide scanning will show inflammatory lesions of bone earlier than do radiographs (Figure 6.43).

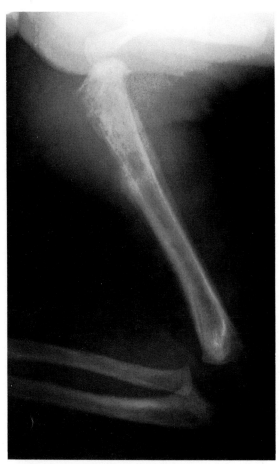

Fig. 6.42 Acute osteomyelitis of humerus, with bone destruction and periosteal reaction.

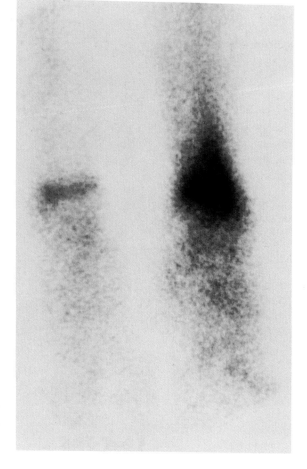

Fig. 6.43 Radionuclide scan of early osteomyelitis of left ankle, showing high uptake of radiopharmaceutical.

Chronic osteomyelitis

This is rarely seen because antibiotics usually abort the disease in its acute phase.

Radiological appearances

1. Areas of destruction of the spongiosa and cortex.

2. Sclerosis of the bone between the areas of destruction.

3. A sheath of new subperiosteal sclerotic bone around and often separated from the original bone (involucrum). There may be gaps in the involucrum (cloacae).

4. Sequestra — fragments of dense, dead bone — may be present. They have lost their blood supply and hence the calcium content remains intact; they appear dense against the surrounding osteoporotic bone (Figure 6.44A).

Brodies abscess

This is a form of chronic osteomyelitis.

Radiological appearances (Figure 6.44B)

1. A small rounded cavity.

2. A surrounding zone of sclerosis.

3. Often a sequestrum in the cavity.

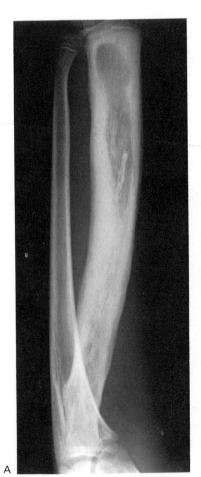
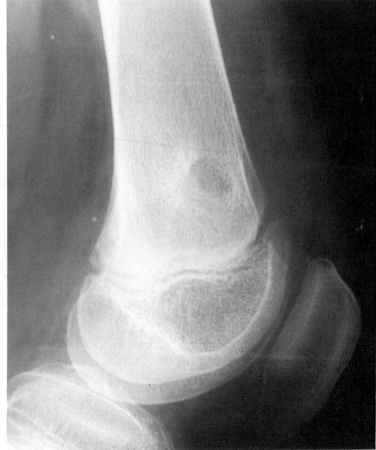

A

B

Fig. 6.44 (A) Chronic osteomyelitis of radius with sequestrum. (B) Brodie's abscess.

Osteomyelitis of the spine

Radiological appearances

1. An area of oesteoporosis and later bone destruction occurs on the disc surface or in the body of a vertebra.

2. Destruction of the disc follows.

3. A spindle-shaped abscess may develop around the spine but, unlike tuberculous abscesses, it does not undergo calcification.

4. With healing, fusion of vertebral bodies may occur.

PYOGENIC ARTHRITIS

The organisms usually responsible are staphylococci, streptococci or pneumococci.

Radiological appearances

Early:

1. Widening of the joint space due to an effusion.

2. Osteoporosis of bones in the area.

Later:

3. Narrowing of the joint space due to cartilage destruction.

4. Destruction of the bones at the joint — this may be massive (Figure 6.45).

Later:

5. With healing the bones recalcify and there may be bony or fibrous ankylosis of the joint.

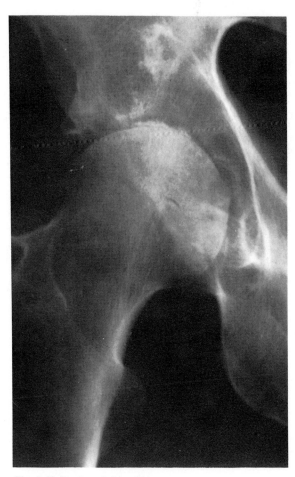

Fig. 6.45 Septic arthritis of hip.

TUBERCULOSIS OF BONE

Long bones

The infection usually commences in the metaphysis of long bones and then spreads to involve the epiphysis. Unlike pyogenic infections the lesion is apparent at the initial examination and periosteal thickening and sequestra are *not* features.

Radiological appearances

1. An area of osteoporosis within which is an area of bone destruction which may be well or ill defined.
2. Little or no periosteal reaction.

Spine

Three sites of infection are commonly described:

1. Anterior part of the disc surface of a vertebral body
2. Anterior surface of the vertebral body
3. Central in the vertebral body.

The anterior part of the disc surface of the vertebral body is the common site and frequently the adjacent surfaces of two vertebrae are involved.

Radiological appearances

1. Disc surface (Figure 6.46)
   (a) Destruction of the anterior edge of the disc surface of the vertebra.
   (b) Rapid destruction of the disc.
   (c) Abscess formation which is manifested by a paravertebral, spindle-shaped, soft tissue mass in the dorsal area and by bulging of the psoas shadow in the lumbar region.
   (d) Spotty calcification may later occur in the abscess (Figure 6.47)
   (e) With healing, the bones regain a well-defined outline but the deformity following the destruction persists.

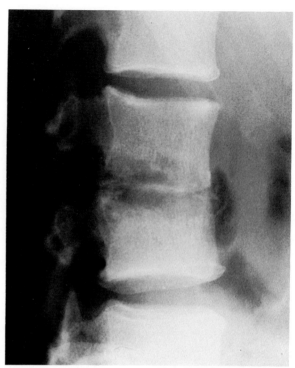

Fig. 6.46 Inflammatory discitis with bone and disc destruction.

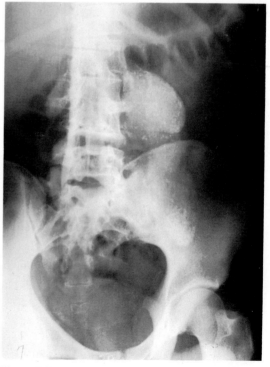

Fig. 6.47 Psoas abscesses due to old spinal tuberculosis.

2. Anterior surface: involvement produces concave erosion of this surface. An abscess may spread up and down the spine under the anterior longitudinal ligament. Aortic pulsation against this abscess may lead to sharply defined concavity of the anterior surfaces of several vertebrae in the mid and lower dorsal area.

3. Central involvement of the vertebral body: this gives an irregular area of destruction which tends to spread to the surface and then resembles either of the other two forms described.

TUBERCULOUS ARTHRITIS

The initial infection may be in the synovial membrane or in a neighbouring bone.

Radiological appearances

1. Synovial infection

Early:

(a) Initially there may be no radiological changes apparent.

Later:

(b) Osteoporosis of the bones in the area.

(c) An effusion which bulges the joint capsule.

Later:

(d) Loss of definition of the bone structure (Figure 6.48).

(e) Loss of joint space due to cartilage destruction may occur later, unlike pyogenic arthritis where it occurs early.

(f) Erosions appear in the bone of the joint surfaces.

(g) In children there may be early maturation of epiphyses due to the hyperaemia.

2. Bone infection. The same sequence of events occurs but there is also a bone lesion present. As the result of modern treatment only the early signs of disease are usually seen.

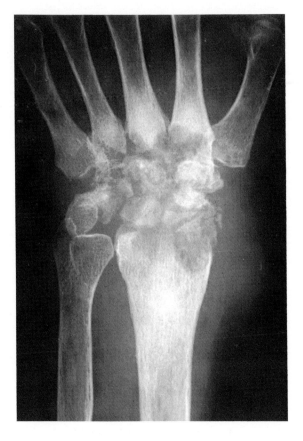

Fig. 6.48 Tuberculosis of wrist, with bone and joint destruction.

THE ARTHRITIDES

RHEUMATOID ARTHRITIS
The small joints of the hands and particularly of the feet are most commonly affected but large joints are not exempt and may be the only areas involved. In the feet changes are most common at the metatarso-phalangeal joints, and in the hands the metacarpo-phalangeal and proximal interphalangeal joints are principally affected, but the distal interphalangeal joints may sometimes show the changes. Involvement of the carpal and wrist joints is common and there may be erosion of the tip of the ulnar styloid process.

Radiological appearances (Figure 6.49)
The changes in small and large joints are very similar.

1. Peri-articular osteoporosis: a common early sign.
2. Erosions: these appear at the margins of the articular surface and later spread across the surface.
3. Joint narrowing: in the early stages there may be widening of the joint space due to an effusion but later there is narrowing of the space due to cartilage destruction.
4. Soft tissue thickening: this forms a spindle-shaped soft tissue shadow around the joint.
5. Cysts: small cyst-like areas may be seen in the subarticular bone of small joints and are probably erosions seen en face. Larger cysts may occur close to large joints.

Complications
1. Secondary osteoarthritis: a common end-result in both large and small joints.
2. Ankylosis: this may be the end result and may be bony or fibrous.
3. Spinal subluxation: rheumatoid may effect the cervical spine. Erosive changes occur at the apophyseal joints and vertebral disc surfaces with narrowing of intervertebral discs. As the result of bone changes and softening of ligaments there may be a forward subluxation of the first on the second cervical vertebra.

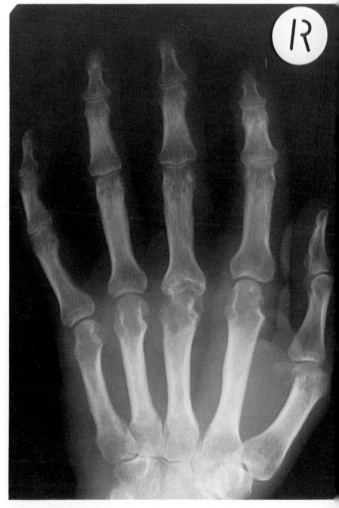

Fig. 6.49 Early rheumatoid arthritis, with peri-articular erosions.

Rheumatoid arthritis in children (Still's disease)

Still's disease is a triad of rheumatoid polyarthritis, enlarged spleen and enlarged lymph nodes. Rheumatoid arthritis produces similar changes in children's joints to those seen in adults, with common involvement of large joints and the cervical spine. Accelerated maturation of ossification centres for epiphyses and sesamoid bones, as the result of hyperaemia, is often a feature. The tubular bones of the hands are often narrow with flared ends (Figure 6.50).

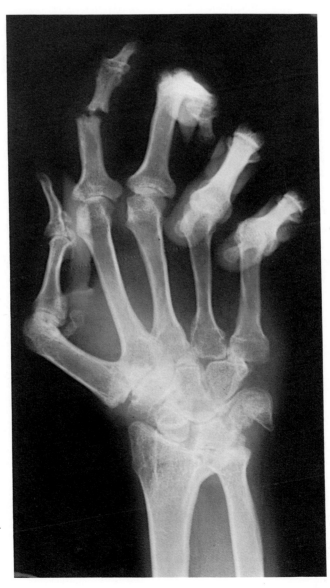

Fig. 6.50 Still's disease.

ANKYLOSING SPONDYLITIS

Radiological appearances (Figure 6.51)

1. Rheumatoid-like changes in the sacro-iliac joints — osteoporosis, erosions, early joint widening and later joint narrowing, followed by sclerosis of bone and often bony ankylosis.

2. New bone is deposited on the concave anterior aspect of vertebral bodies and as a result the body assumes a square shape.

3. Ossification of the paraspinal ligaments which produces the typical 'bamboo spine'.

PSORIATIC ARTHRITIS

This condition may affect the hands in cases of psoriasis. The changes are similar to those of rheumatoid arthritis but tend to affect the distal rather than the proximal interphalangeal joints. Absorption of the terminal tufts of the distal phalanges and an absence of osteoporosis are common features.

OSTEOARTHRITIS

Osteoarthritis is a degenerative condition and may be primary, arising in a normal joint, or secondary, arising in a joint previously damaged by trauma or disease. The changes develop slowly but in an established case a number of changes are seen.

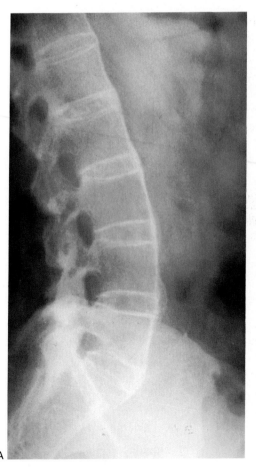
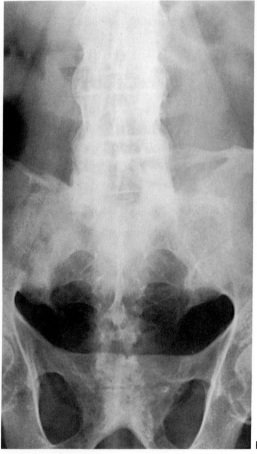

A   B

Fig. 6.51 Lateral (A) and AP (B) views of lumbo-sacral spine in ankylosing spondylitis. Note fusion of vertebrae, sacro-iliac joints, and symphysis pubis.

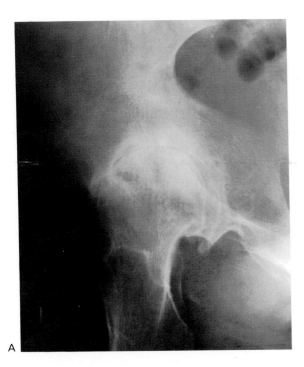

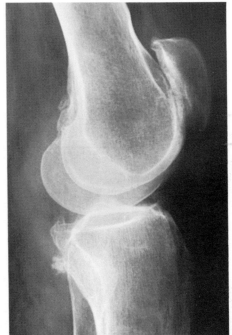

Radiological appearances (Figure 6.52)

1. Joint space narrowing: the result of degeneration of cartilage.

2. Sclerosis: the joint surfaces are sclerotic.

3. Pseudocysts: cyst-like spaces develop in the subarticular bone.

4. Osteophytes: bony spurs which usually develop at the margins of the articular surfaces, but which at the knee joint first develop at the tibial spine and patella.

5. Loose bodies: these may develop from detached osteophytes or from fragments of degenerating cartilage.

6. New bone: periosteal new bone formation on the under surface of the femoral neck and within the acetabulum are commonly seen in osteoarthritis of the hip.

True osteoarthritic changes occur at the apophyseal joints in the spine. The condition of disc narrowing and osteophytes on the margins of vertebral bodies is not a true osteoarthritis but a condition called spondylosis, which is usually secondary to disc degeneration. Osteophytes in the region of neural foramina may irritate nerve roots and those on the dorsal aspect of the body may affect the spinal cord.

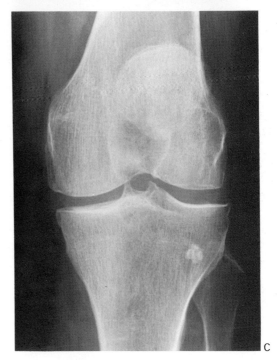

Fig. 6.52 (A) Osteoarthritis of hip.
(B) and (C) AP and lateral views of early osteoarthritis of knee.

GOUT

Although a metabolic disease, gout is best considered in this section because joint changes are a cardinal feature.

Radiological appearances (Figure 6.53)

1. Erosions: these are well-defined areas in the cortex of bones close to a joint. They are better defined than the erosions of rheumatoid arthritis and tend to spread along the bone away from the joint as well as eroding the joint surface. They are due to deposits of sodium biurate.

2. Joint space narrowing: this occurs late in the disease.

3. Tophi: eccentric soft tissue swellings in the region of the joint which may occasionally calcify and are due to urate deposits.

Differential diagnosis

Difficulty may sometimes be experienced in differentiating gout and rheumatoid arthritis but the following points may help.

1. Erosions: these are better defined and tend to spread along the shaft in gout.

2. Soft tissue swelling: fusiform in rheumatoid arthritis and eccentric in gout.

3. Interphalangeal joints: gout tends to involve the distal, and rheumatoid the proximal, joints.

4. Tophi: if calcified, these are characteristic of gout.

5. Blood chemistry: the serum uric acid is raised in gout.

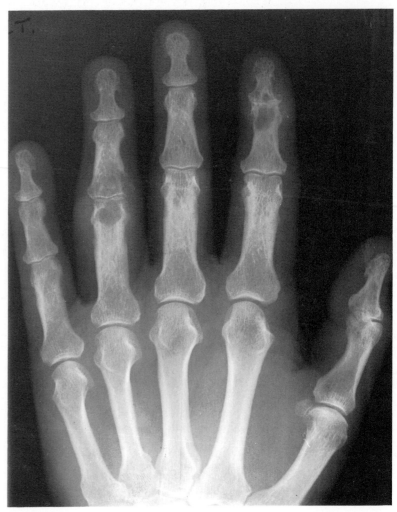

Fig. 6.53 Gout involving hand with bone destruction and early tophi.

NEUROPATHIC JOINTS

As the result of diminished pain sense, trauma to a joint may go unnoticed by the patient. Repeated traumatic episodes eventually lead to marked disorganization and degeneration of the joint. The predisposing conditions are:

1. Diabetic neuropathy, which affects the small joints of the feet.

2. Leprosy, mostly affecting the small joints of the hands and feet.

3. Syringomyelia, affecting the large joints of the shoulder and arm.

4. Neurosyphilis, which affects the large joints of the leg and arm, particularly the knee joint.

5. Congenital absence of pain sense, which produces changes particularly of the lower limb in children.

6. Spina bifida, in which some cases exhibit diminished pain sense in the lower limbs.

7. Paralysed limbs, whereby neuropathic joints may develop if pain sense is diminished.

Radiological appearances (Figure 6.54)

1. Destruction of the joint surfaces: the destruction may be generalized or may involve only a portion of the joint surface, sometimes with a sharply defined straight margin between the area of destruction and the remainder of the bone.

2. Loose bodies: fragments of detached bone may lie free within the joint.

3. Joint space narrowing: this results from the destruction of bone and articular cartilage.

4. Sclerosis: this may be present in the opposing bones of the joint.

5. Dislocation: marked destruction of the joint may sometimes allow a dislocation to occur.

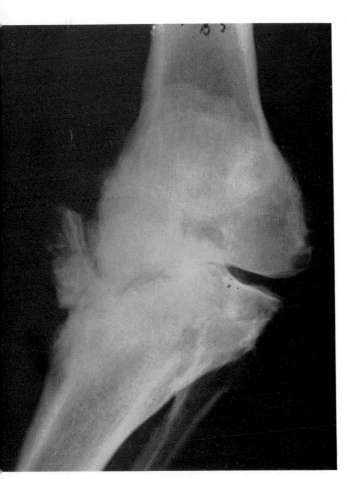

Fig. 6.54 Neuropathic knee joint with sclerosis, destruction, and calcified debris.

BONE TUMOURS

Bone tumours are rare. They may arise from the cells of bone, cartilage, connective tissue, synovium, marrow, blood vessels or nerves. They are thus a diverse group; the details of which are beyond the scope of this text in which only a few examples of the less uncommon types are considered.

However, because of the young age group most commonly affected and the hazard of possible malignant change they merit a greater general consideration than their incidence would suggest. In a given case two prime decisions must be attempted:

1. Is the lesion due to a bone tumour?
2. If it is a tumour is it benign or malignant?

The answers may be easy or very difficult even with the essential cooperation of clinician, radiologist and pathologist. Factors such as the age and sex of the patient and clinical history and findings are often as relevant as the radiological appearances.

IS THE LESION A BONE TUMOUR?
This question arises most often in the case of a young person presenting with a low grade fever, some swelling and tenderness over a bone and a radiograph showing periosteal reaction and bone destruction in the area. All of these findings can be common to acute osteomyelitis and bone sarcoma. The response to antibiotics will probably give the answer but this takes time.

Examination of the soft tissue planes on the radiograph may help, since in cases of infection they tend to be obliterated by oedema whereas with an early tumour they are usually well defined.

IS THE TUMOUR BENIGN OR MALIGNANT?
There are some broad radiological criteria which may help.

Benign tumours
1. The lesion commonly has a well-defined margin.
2. A zone of sclerosis often surrounds the lesion.

Malignant tumours
1. The margin of the lesion is usually ill defined.
2. A break in the overlying cortex, especially if there is an associated soft tissue mass, is strongly suggestive of malignancy.
3. Periosteal reaction such as elevation or onion layering and the 'sunray' radiating spicules sometimes seen are *not* specific to bone tumours. If they occur where there is a degree of certainty that the lesion is a tumour they are, however, suggestive of malignancy.

BENIGN TUMOURS

Simple bone cyst
They are always solitary and most common at the proximal ends of the humerus, tibia and femur. They usually present as a pathological fracture in childhood. They develop first in the metaphysis but, as the bone grows, come to lie further down the shaft.

Radiological appearances (Figure 6.55)
A well-defined area of radiolucency surrounded by a thin zone of sclerosis. Thinning of the overlying cortex is common.

Chondroma
The most common sites are the tubular bones of the hands, but they are not uncommon in other bones. All, particularly those in flat bones, are potentially malignant and periosteal reaction or change in the radiological appearance strongly suggests malignant change. It is uncommon, however, for malignant change to occur in lesions in the hands and feet.

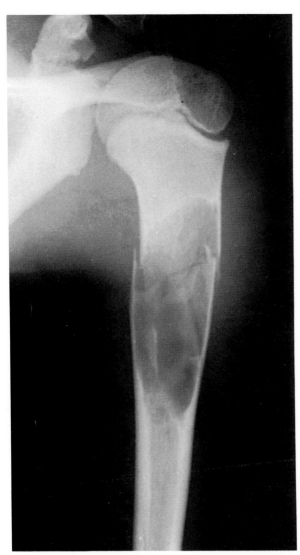

Fig. 6.55 Simple bone cyst of humerus, with fracture.

Radiological appearances (Figure 6.56)

1. A well-defined area of translucency in the bone.

2. In the hands and feet the cortex is often thinned and expanded.

3. Flecks of calcification in the area of translucency are common.

4. In long bones: (a) if eccentrically placed they thin the cortex from within; (b) usually sharply defined; (c) sclerosis in the surrounding bone is common.

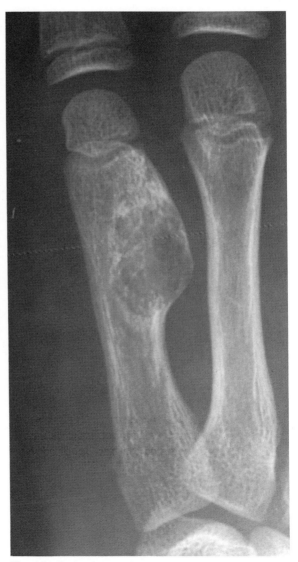

Fig. 6.56 Enchondroma of metacarpal.

Multiple enchondromata

There are enchondromata in many bones (Figure 6.57); the condition is associated with dwarfism.

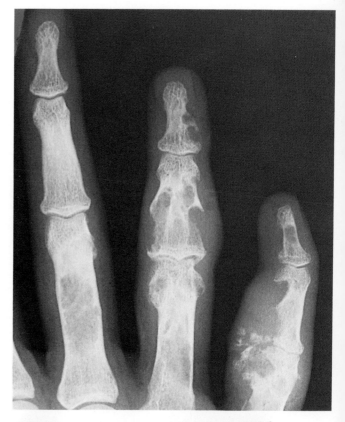

Fig. 6.57 Multiple enchondromata of phalanges.

Osteochondroma

This usually arises from the metaphysis of a long bone and is formed by cortical and cancellous bone with a cartilage cap. It may be flat or pedunculated and pointing away from the epiphysis (Figure 6.58). The cartilage cap may sometimes undergo malignant change.

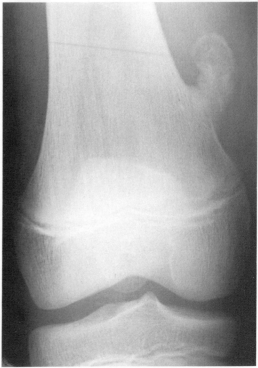

Fig. 6.58 Osteochondroma of lower end of femur.

Osteid osteoma

The most common sites are the femur and tibia but it may occur in any bone except the skull. It occurs mostly in males under 30 years.

Radiological appearances (Figure 6.59)

1. An area of radiolucency within which may be a central density. This complex is called the nidus.

2. A zone of sclerosis, most marked in cortical lesions, may surround the translucent area.

3. If sclerosis is marked, tomography may help to show the nidus.

Differential diagnosis

Osteoid osteoma must be distinguished from a Brodie's abscess. The abscess may have a sequestrum and cloacae which help in diferentiation.

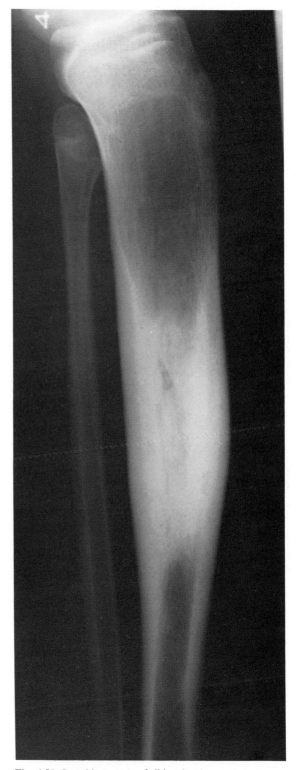

Fig. 6.59 Osteoid osteoma of tibia, showing central nidus.

Benign chondroblastoma

These usually arise in the epiphysis of a long
bone and then cross to the metaphysis. They are
most common at the upper end of the humerus.
Males in the second decade are particularly
affected.

Radiological appearances (Figure 6.60)

1. An area of radiolucency involving the
epiphysis more than the metaphysis.

2. The margin is well defined with a thin
zone of sclerosis.

3. There may be flecks of calcification
present.

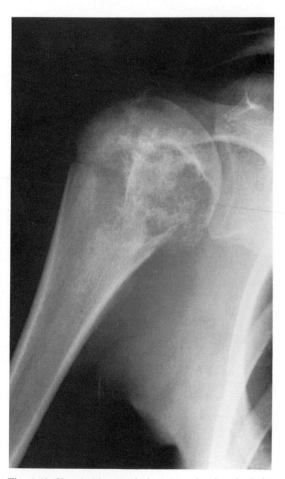

Fig. 6.60 Chondroblastoma in humerus, showing the lesion
crossing the epiphyseal line.

MALIGNANT TUMOURS

Metastases

It is always important to remember that the
most common malignant bone tumour over the
age of 40 years is a metastasis. The most
common sites are the spine, pelvis, ribs, skull,
humerus and femur; they rarely occur below the
elbow or knee. The most common metastases
arise from kidney, breast, lung, prostate and
colon. In children they are commonly from a
neuroblastoma before the age of 5, and from
Ewing's tumour at a later age. Metastases which
expand bone arise from kidney, thyroid and
lung.

Radiological appearances

1. The vast majority are osteolytic (Figure
6.61).

2. There is no significant periosteal reaction.

3. Breast metastases are mostly osteolytic, a
few are osteoblastic and some are mixed.
Prostatic metastases are mostly osteoblastic and
occur particularly in the pelvis and spine (Figure
6.62). Kidney metastases are osteolytic, expansile
and often solitary. Lung metastases are mostly
osteolytic.

4. Radionuclide bone scanning may show
metastases before they are visible on plain
radiography (Figure 6.63).

Differential diagnosis

Difficulty may be experienced in differentiating
multiple metastases and the lesions of multiple
myeloma. Bence Jones protein is present in the
urine in 60% of cases of multiple myeloma.

With prostatic metastases the serum acid
phosphatase is raised, but in Paget's disease,
with which prostatic metastases may be
confused, the serum alkaline phosphatase is
markedly elevated.

Aneurysmal bone cyst

The majority are in long bones, but no bone is
exempt. They occur most frequently in the
second and third decades; radiotherapy is
curative.

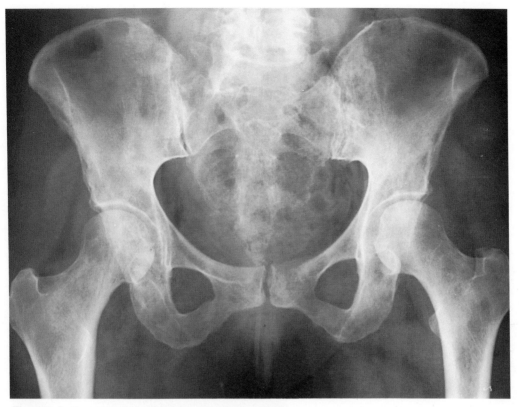

Fig. 6.61 Lytic metastases from carcinoma of breast.

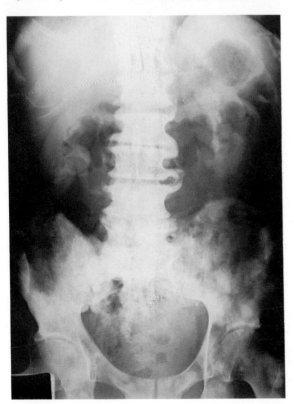

Radiological appearances

1. A cystic area usually eccentrically placed in a long bone.

2. The cortex is eroded and expanded and may be destroyed.

3. There is a sharply defined sclerotic inner margin.

4. Growth is usually slow but may be rapid.

Aneurysmal bone cyst must be distinguished from a giant cell tumour, which usually occurs in an older age after the epiphyses have closed, and which has a rather ill-defined endosteal margin.

Fig. 6.62 Sclerotic metastases from carcinoma of prostate.

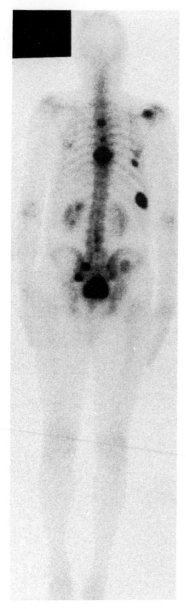

Fig. 6.63 Radionuclide bone scan showing neoplastic metastases

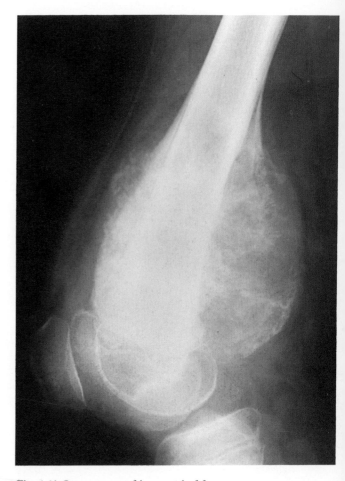

Fig. 6.64 Osteosarcoma of lower end of femur.

Osteosarcoma (osteogenic sarcoma)

This is the most common primary malignant bone tumour. It has a peak incidence between 10 and 25 years and a further peak over the age of 50 when it complicates Paget's disease. The serum alkaline phosphatase is raised, indicating active osteoid formation.

Radiological appearances (Figure 6.64)

1. Usually sited in the metaphysis of a long bone, especially near the knee.

2. The epiphyseal plate usually limits spread towards the knee until late in the process.

3. It is usually a destructive lesion but there is usually some dense irregular new bone formation present. Sometimes the bone is very dense with little or no evidence of destruction or periosteal reaction.

4. Periosteal reaction produces layers of bone density, parallel to the shaft (onion layering).

5. The cortex ultimately becomes eroded and a soft tissue mass forms.

6. The new periosteal bone becomes eroded centrally leaving triangular areas of new bone at the edges (Codman's triangle).

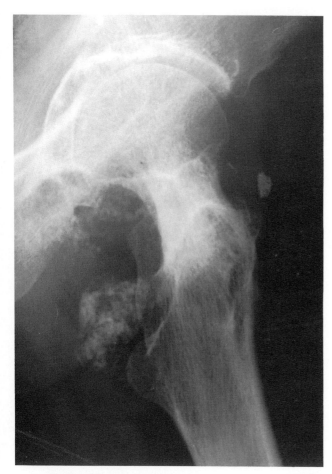

Fig. 6.65 Chondrosarcoma of upper end of femur, showing cartilage calcification.

7. Sometimes spicules of new bone radiate out from the lesion to give the sunray appearance.

It is worth reiterating that Codman's triangle and the sunray appearance do not necessarily indicate malignancy. The sunray appearance can also be seen in haemangioma, meningioma, Ewing's tumour, metastases and pyogenic osteomyelitis, and is not characteristic of osteosarcoma.

Paget's sarcoma
A rare complication of Paget's disease, it may sometimes be multifocal and is usually destructive, although sometimes there is also new bone formation.

Irradiation sarcoma
This usually occurs many years after irradiation of a bone; its appearances are the same as osteosarcoma.

Chondrosarcoma
Unlike osteosarcoma, chondrosarcoma occurs most commonly in middle age. The tumour may arise *de novo* or develop from a pre-existing cartilage tumour such as an enchondroma or an osteochondroma so that in relation to the bone it may be centrally or peripherally placed. Any change in the radiological appearance of a cartilage tumour should be viewed with suspicion that malignant change has occurred.

Central chondrosarcoma are most common in the shafts of the femur and tibia, but also occur in flat bones such as the pelvis, ribs and skull.

Radiological appearances
Long bones:
1. An area of bone destruction within the area of which there are often flecks of calcification.
2. There may be a surrounding zone of bone sclerosis.
3. The bone may be expanded and the overlying cortex breached.
4. Periosteal reaction is usually not a prominent feature.
5. There may be a soft tissue mass present due to tumour.

Flat bones:
There may only be an area of bone destruction with little or no areas of calcification.

In the case of peripheral chondrosarcoma, clinically there may be a history of a recent increase in size of a bony lump.

Radiological appearances (Figure 6.65)
1. The margins of an osteochondroma may be irregular.
2. There may be flecks of calcification in the neighbouring soft tissues.

Giant cell tumour

This tumour is most common in the region of the knee joint, the distal end of the radius, and the upper end of humerus. The sacrum is the usual site if the spine is involved. The majority occur between 20 and 40 years of age. They are locally malignant.

Radiological appearances (Figure 6.66)

1. An area of translucency extending to the articular surface develops in the end of a long bone and has a multi-locular appearance.

2. The endosteal margin is hazy.

3. Tends to be eccentrically placed and thins and expands the cortex.

4. There is no periosteal reaction.

5. The cortex may be destroyed with formation of a soft tissue mass.

6. Suspect malignant change if the tumour grows rapidly and there is increased cortical destruction.

Differential diagnosis

1. Simple cyst — younger age group.

2. Aneurysmal bone cyst — not usually subarticular.

Ewing's sarcoma

Common in the mid-shaft of long bones but any bone can be involved and 50% of cases occur in flat bones in particular in the pelvis. The peak incidence is between 10 and 20 years.

Radiological appearances (Figure 6.67)

Similar to osteosarcoma with periosteal thickening usually being a prominent feature. It is more commonly situated in the mid-shaft of a long bone than is osteosarcoma.

Differential diagnosis

1. Osteomyelitis — this may be difficult to distinguish from a Ewing's sarcoma in the early stages, although onion-layering of the periosteal reaction, if present, is more suggestive of tumour than infection.

2. Eosinophilic granuloma may mimic the appearances.

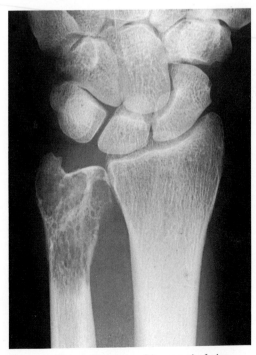

Fig. 6.66 Giant cell tumour of lower end of ulna.

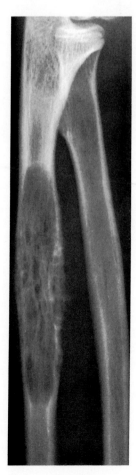

Fig. 6.67 Ewing's tumour of ulna, with destruction and periosteal reaction.

BONE CHANGES IN HAEMOPOIETIC DISORDERS AND RETICULO-ENDOTHELIAL DISORDERS

In infancy the red blood cell forming marrow extends throughout the whole skeleton. By late adolescence the extent of this marrow has shrunk and is confined to the spine, skull, flat bones and proximal ends of the femora and humeri. Chronic haemolytic anaemias, which are congenital, cause an increase in the extent of this marrow and radiological changes become apparent in the bones. These changes are widening of the spongiosa, coarse trabecular pattern, and thinning of the cortex (Figure 6.68).

The group includes thalassaemia (Cooley's anaemia) which is most common in Mediterranean people and their descendents, and sickle cell anaemia which is almost completely confined to negroes.

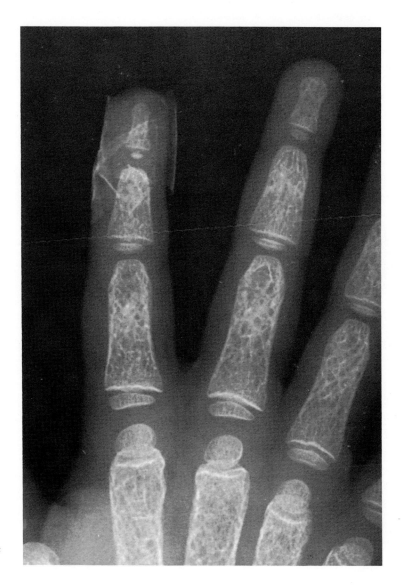

Fig. 6.68 Thallassaemia, with medullary widening and coarse trabeculation.

PLASMOCYTOMA AND MULTIPLE MYELOMA

A malignant neoplasm arising from marrow cells, particularly in bones where haemopoiesis is occurring — spine, pelvis, ribs, femoral and humeral shafts. It may be solitary — plasmocytoma — or multicentric. It is rare before the age of 40. Bence Jones proteinuria is present in 60% of cases and is pathognomonic.

Radiological appearances
1. Solitary lesion: a lucent, markedly expanding area in bone.
2. Multiple lesions (Figure 6.69)
   (a) Osteoporosis of the skeleton, alone or with many lytic lesions.
   (b) Well-defined lytic areas scattered throughout the bones where haemopoiesis is occurring.
   (c) Vertebral bodies may be collapsed but the vertebral appendages are not affected until late in the disease.

Differential diagnosis
1. Metastases. Usually not as well-defined as myelomatous lesions and tend not to involve the mandible.
2. Hyerparathyroidism. Multiple 'brown tumours' may simulate myelomatous deposits.

Sternal marrow biopsy will differentiate myelomatous from other lesions.

Because proteinaceous material may block the renal collecting system, excretory pyelography has been thought to be contraindicated, but evidence exists that the diatrizoate compounds in current use are relatively safe.

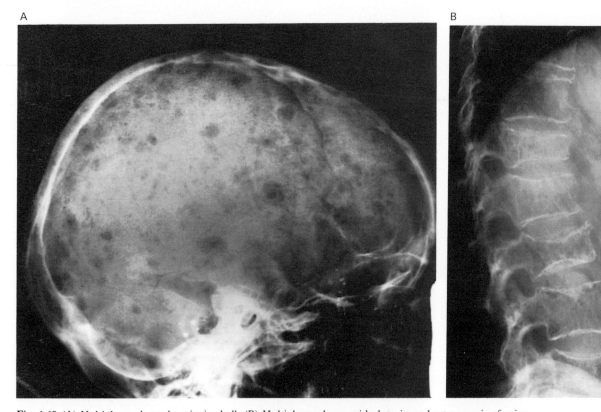

A   B

Fig. 6.69 (A) Multiple myeloma deposits in skull. (B) Multiple myeloma, with deposits and osteoporosis of spine.

LEUKAEMIA

Radiological appearances

1. Children. The leukaemia is usually acute and skeletal changes are present in approximately 50% of cases: (a) diffuse osteoporosis; (b) radiolucent bands in the diaphyses of long bones, particularly in the knee area; (c) small radiolucent defects in bones; (d) periosteal thickening in long bones.

2. Adults. In acute leukaemia death usually precedes skeletal changes. In the chronic form bone changes are infrequent radiologically but the following may be seen: (a) generalized osteoporosis — the most common finding; (b) poorly defined areas of destruction which may be discrete or confluent and may cause vertebral collapse.

LYMPHADENOMA (HODGKIN'S DISEASE)

Most lesions are found in the red bone marrow areas so that the spine, thoracic cage and pelvis are the common sites.

Radiological appearances

There are three main types of change seen:

1. Osteolytic areas with thinning and expansion of the overlying cortex seen particularly in the ribs, the proximal ends of the humeri and femora, and the vertebrae.

2. Sclerosis of bone, but unlike Paget's disease there is no expansion of bone. It is most commonly seen in vertebral bodies and pelvis. A single dense vertebral body in a young person is strongly suggestive of lymphadenoma.

3. Mixed sclerosing and osteolytic types, seen most commonly in the pelvis.

LYMPHOSARCOMA

Radiological appearances

The bone changes are very similar to osteolytic Hodgkin's disease but with a much faster progression; they also tend to occur in the red marrow areas.

HISTIOCYTOSIS X

There are three forms of this disease.

Eosinophilic granuloma

This commonly affects children and young adults and is most common in males. Long bones are affected but it is more common in the skull, pelvis and spine.

Radiological appearances (Figure 6.70)

1. Usually a single fairly small area of bone destruction with a well-defined, bevelled edge.

2. Surrounding sclerosis may be present in lesions which are healing.

3. There may be slight expansion of bone and some thickening of the overlying periosteum in long bones.

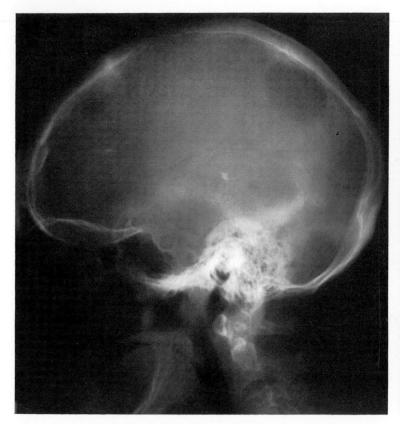

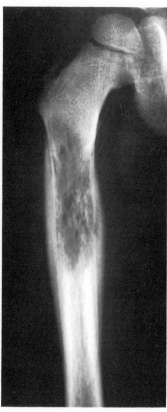

Fig. 6.70 (A) Eosinophilic granuloma involving skull.
(B) Eosinophilic granuloma of femur,
with destruction and reaction.

4. The lesions are usually solitary but as one undergoes spontaneous healing another may appear.

5. Spontaneous regression is not uncommon.

6. In the spine there may be marked collapse and flattening of a vertebral body but this, too, can return to a normal appearance.

Hand–Schuller–Christian disease (xanthomatosis)

This is most common in young children.

Radiological appearances

The changes are the same as those in eosinophilic granuloma but tend to be multiple and to affect particularly the flat bones. In the skull the areas may fuse to produce a large irregular osteolytic area — the map skull.

Letterer–Siwe disease

This condition mostly occurs before 2 years and is usually fatal. It is associated with severe clinical symptoms.

Radiological appearances

There may be no bone changes or there may be multiple, scattered, rather ill-defined areas of destruction in bones where haemopoiesis is occurring.

HAEMOPHILIA

Haemophilia occurs principally in males and haemorrhage into joints as the result of mild trauma is common.

Radiological appearances

1. Joint changes (Figure 6.71). Haemorrhages into joints, particularly the knee and elbow, are followed by organization of the blood in the joint which produces a local hyperaemia. The repeated haemarthroses and the chronic hyperaemia lead to: (a) osteoporosis of the bones at the joints; (b) enlarged epiphyses which tend to be square rather than rounded; (c) loss of joint space due to cartilage destruction; (d) sclerosis of joint surfaces; (e) enlargement of the intercondylar notch when the knee is affected.

2. Bone changes. Haemorrhage into the bone produces cystic areas near joints (Figure 6.72).

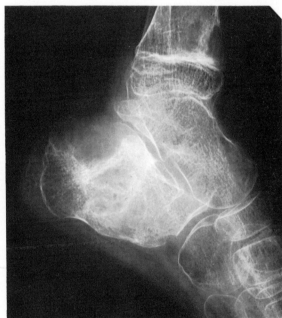

Fig. 6.72 Haemophilia with haemorrhages involving the os calcis.

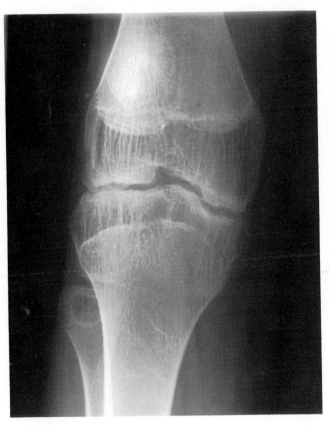

Fig. 6.71 Haemophilic knee, with bone overgrowth and joint damage.

ENDOCRINE AND METABOLIC BONE DISEASE

PRIMARY HYPERPARATHYROIDISM

This results from a parathyroid tumour which produces excessive quantities of parathormone which inhibits absorption of phosphorous by the renal tubules with resulting elevation of the blood and urine calcium. Calcium removed from bones is responsible for the high blood calcium levels. Renal calculi and nephrocalcinosis are common, due to the high urine calcium and phosphate levels. Skeletal changes are present in approximately one-third of cases.

Radiological appearances

1. Subperiosteal erosion is diagnostic (Figure 6.73). It is best seen in the bones of the fingers and appears as tiny holes on the surface of the cortex which give a lace-like border to the bones. Loss of the lamina dura around the teeth is common, but this is also seen in Paget's disease, myelomatosis and osteoporotic conditions.

2. Brown tumours. Well-defined, thin-walled cysts which if large enough will cause expansion of the bone. They may be single or multiple and may be multi-locular.

3. Cortical changes include thickening , with reduction in the width of the marrow cavity and widespread tiny elliptical holes in the cortex. In the skull these holes produce the typical 'pepper pot' appearance.

4. Generalized osteoporosis of the skeleton may be seen late in the disease.

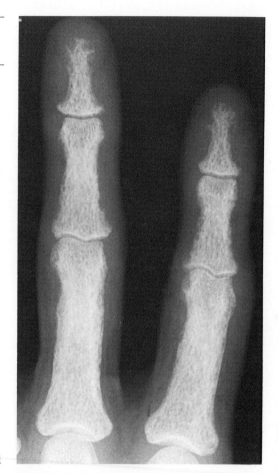

Fig. 6.73 Hand in hyperparathyroidism, with subperiosteal bone resorption.

SECONDARY HYPERPARATHYROIDISM

The common cause of this condition is renal failure due to chronic pyelonephritis and less commonly to chronic glomerulonephritis. The resulting disordered biochemistry exerts a demand for calcium which comes from the bone, in association with hyperplasia of the parathyroids.

Radiological appearances

The changes are similar to those of primary hyperparathyroidism except that 'brown tumours' and nephrocalcinosis are less common. However, ectopic soft tissue and vascular calcification is common.

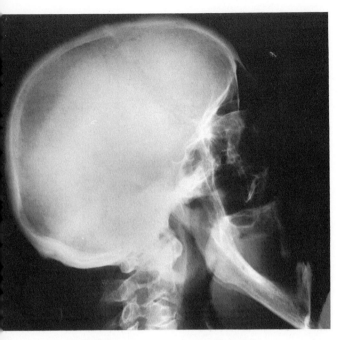

Fig. 6.74 Acromegaly: lateral view of skull.

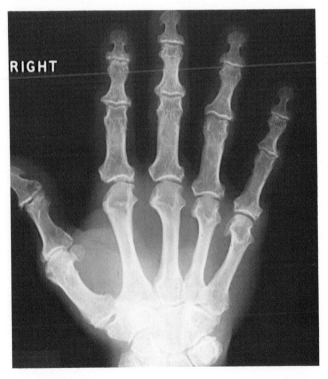

Fig. 6.75 Acromegaly causing bone and joint overgrowth in hand.

HYPERPITUITARISM

An eosinophilic adenoma produces an excess of growth hormone which results in the production of large thick bones with prominent muscular attachments. When it occurs before growth stops the result is gigantism, and after growth stops acromegaly results.

Acromegaly

The skull shows enlargement of the pituitary fossa, the paranasal air sinuses and mastoid air cells (Figure 6.74). The mandible is large and juts out.

Vertebral bodies are enlarged and in the hands and feet there is enlargement of the digital tufts, widening of joint spaces, and thickening of the soft tissues (Figure 6.75). The long bones show very prominent muscular attachments.

Cushing's disease

This results from adrenal cortical hyperactivity resulting in excessive production of cortisone and hydrocortisone and produces the following:

1. Generalized osteoporosis
2. In young people there is delay in skeletal maturation.

HYPOPITUITARISM

This produces dwarfism, with delay in the appearance and fusion of epiphyseal centres, delayed closure of cranial sutures, and delayed dentition.

HYPOTHYROIDISM
Hypothyroidism results in cretinism in infants.

Radiological appearances
1. Marked delay in dentition, closure of cranial sutures and appearance of ossific centres throughout the skeleton.
2. Epiphyses often have multiple centres of ossification (Figure 6.76).

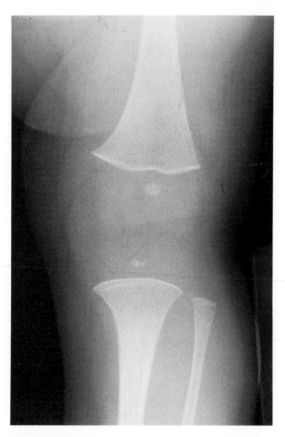

Fig. 6.76 Cretinism in a neonate. Note stippled epiphyses.

VITAMIN RELATED BONE DISEASE

An understanding of the zones at the end of a normal growing bone is necessary to appreciate the changes seen in this region in vitamin related bone disease. There are three zones (Figure 6.77).
1. A layer of cartilage which is radiolucent.
2. A dense band due to provisional calcification of cartilage.
3. A zone where the calcified cartilage is being converted to bone.

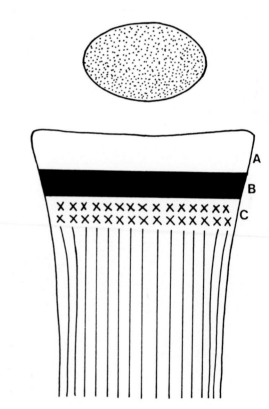

Fig. 6.77 Diagram of growing end of bone:
(A) cartilage;
(B) zone of provisional calcification;
(C) bone formation.

VITAMIN D DEFICIENCY
This produces rickets before skeletal maturation, and osteomalacia in adults.

Rickets

There are two forms of rickets, dependent on the cause.

1. Ordinary rickets is due to lack of vitamin D in the diet, resistance to vitamin D, or failure of absorption of calcium and vitamin D from the intestine in small bowel disease such as steatorrhoea.

2. Renal rickets is due to metabolic upsets, which affect the levels of calcium and phosphorous in the blood and urine, such as chronic renal failure, renal tubular acidosis, and idiopathic hypercalcuria. The basic abnormality is a failure of cartilage and newly formed bone to calcify and this is accompanied by demineralization of normal bone formed before the onset of rickets. The changes are best seen at the ends of long bones.

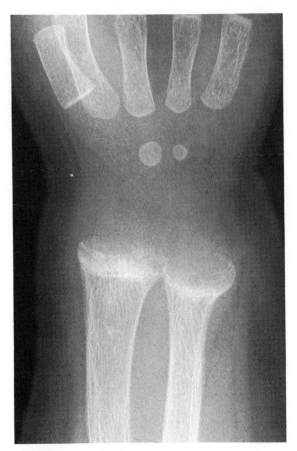

Fig. 6.78 Rickets showing widening of epiphyseal plates, and splaying of metaphyses.

Radiological apperances (Figure 6.78)
Early:

1. The zone of provisional calcification at the end of long bones is narrowed or absent.

2. The gap between the epiphyseal ossification centre and the calcified shaft of the bone is increased.

3. The metaphysis is ragged in contour and often concave.

Later:

4. The shafts of the bones become osteoporotic and may fracture or, with weight-bearing, they may bend.

5. Looser's zones (see 'Osteomalacia', below) may develop in the shaft.

6. Epiphyseal ossification centres appear late and are small and hazy in outline.

With treatment, the new bone formed at the metaphysis and under the periosteum becomes calcified and radiographs then reveal deformities due to failure of bone moulding. If treatment is adequate the bones finally return to normal.

Osteomalacia

This results from a lack of calcium for bone formation. The major causes are inadequate calcium intake, excessive loss of calcium in renal disease, and poor absorption of vitamin D in conditions causing malabsorption, such as steatorrhoea and Crohn's disease.

Radiological appearances

1. There is a generalized loss of calcium from the skeleton.

2. Pseudo-fractures (Looser's zones) — a narrow band of translucency across the shaft of a bone. There may be sclerosis bounding this band if treatment has commenced.

3. Later the bones have a thin cortex and absent trabecular pattern, the vertebral bodies are biconcave (fish vertebrae) with wide intervertebral discs. The pelvis is contracted due to protrusion of the acetabuli and sacrum into the pelvic cavity. The femora are bowed.

VITAMIN C DEFICIENCY (SCURVY)

Inadequate intake of vitamin C produces scurvy, in which there is retarded osteoblastic activity and hence a failure of bone formation. *In infants the changes do not tend to occur before 5 months.*

Radiological appearances (Figure 6.79)
1. The bones are thin and have little or no trabecular pattern.
2. The zone of provisional calcification is widened.
3. There is a zone of osteoporosis on the diaphyseal side of the zone of provisional calcification.
4. The ossific centres of the epiphyses are surrounded by a zone of increased density.
5. Fracture through the osteoporotic zone at the diaphysis is common and the thick zone of provisional calcification becomes impacted on the shaft and juts out laterally — 'Pelkan's spurs'.
6. Subperiosteal haemorrhages occur and become apparent when they calcify.
7. With healing the band of sclerosis may persist and move away from the joint along the shaft.

Differential diagnosis
1. Still's disease: there is no zone of density present.
2. Battered baby: undamaged bones do not show the typical metaphyseal changes of scurvy.

HYPERVITAMINOSIS D

This produces hypercalcaemia, which results in:
1. Dense bands in the metaphyses in children.
2. Metastatic calcification in areas such as the kidney, peri-articular tissue and the vascular system.

Differential diagnosis

In addition to hypervitaminosis D, dense bands may be seen in the metaphysis in heavy metal poisoning such as lead poisoning, and similar lines sometimes associated with a line of rarefaction may be seen in hypothyroidism, syphilis, and leukaemia in children.

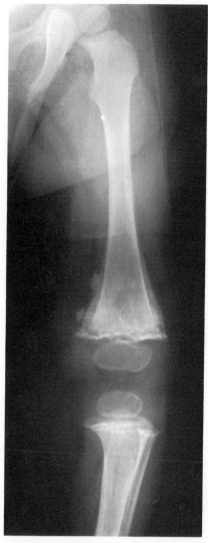

Fig. 6.79 Scurvy, showing dense zones of provisional calcification, Pelken's spurs, and subperiosteal haemorrhage commencing to calcify.

7 The Nervous System

Imaging of the nervous system involves principally the central nervous system, including the brain and its coverings and the eye. The spine, spinal cord and nerve roots may also be imaged, but peripheral nerves are as yet not amenable to imaging.

Brain and skull

Methods of investigation

Plain radiographs
The bony structures of the skull, as well as physiological and pathological intracranial calcifications, are shown.

Computerized tomography (CT)
CT is undoubtedly the most useful of the current modalities (Figure 7.1).

Angiography
Angiography (Figure 7.2) has been largely supplanted by CT but it is still of use to show the details of vascular lesions such as berry aneurysms, arteriovenous malformations and arterial stenoses. The advent of low-dose digital subtraction angiography (page 5) may well lead to extension of the use of the technique (Fig 7.3).

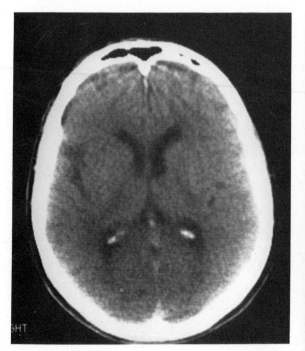

Fig. 7.1 Normal CT scan of brain at level of lateral ventricles.

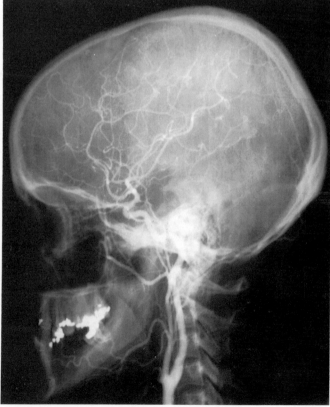

Fig. 7.2 Normal carotid angiogram, lateral projection.

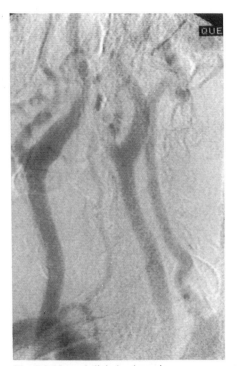

Fig. 7.3 Normal digital subtraction angiogram of cervical vessels.

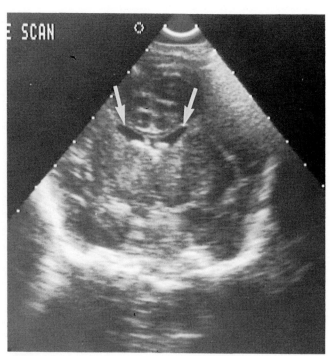

Fig. 7.4 Normal ultrasound of neonatal brain. Lateral ventricles (→).

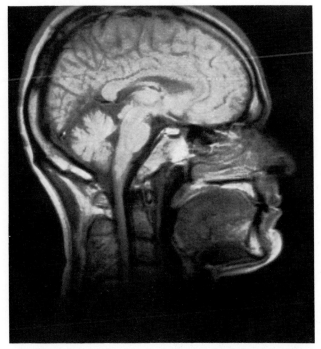

Fig. 7.5 Normal magnetic resonance image of brain, midline sagittal section (Philips Gyroscan, by courtesy of Philips Medical Systems Div, Eindhoven, The Netherlands).

Ultrasound

The prime use of ultrasound is in infants in whom the open fontanelles and thin vault provide adequate acoustic windows (Figure 7.4). Over the age of approximately 2 years ultrasound cannot be used except to localize the midline structures.

Radionuclide scan

Although to a great extent replaced by CT, radionuclide scanning is still used to study localized pathological processes such as infarcts in the brain.

Magnetic resonance imaging (MRI)

This shows great promise in displaying soft tissue anatomy and chemical pathology, e.g. demyelinating diseases, better than CT (Figure 7.5). The ultimate place of the method has yet to emerge.

LESIONS OF BRAIN AND SKULL

CONGENITAL ABNORMALITIES

These are frequently associated with lesions of the spine and spinal cord and will be considered in that section.

TRAUMA

Central nervous system trauma is very common, especially in relation to road traffic accidents, and imaging investigations are an integral part of clinical management.

Fractured skull

Although in itself it is of relatively little importance, a fracture may be indicative of the force and localization of an injury. Fractures may be either fissure or depressed. In either case, extension across the line of the meningeal vessels suggests the possibility of extradural haemorrhage. Plain radiographs are useful in detecting vault fractures (see 'Skull fractures', page 159), but fractures of the skull base are much more difficult to demonstrate, even with conventional or computerized tomography.

Dural tears

These may give rise to cerebrospinal fluid leaks through the ear (fractured petrous temporal) or nose (fractured sinus or cribriform plate). Location of the fracture may require radionuclide cerebrospinal fluid scanning in addition to plain films and possibly CT.

Contusions and lacerations of the brain

These may be directly associated with the site of trauma, but may also be removed or contra-coup. Bleeding into the brain or subarachnoid space may be clearly seen on CT or MRI, and these investigations can be of major prognostic importance (Figure 7.6).

The pineal gland is situated in the midline of the brain in the coronal plane, is calcified in 30% of adults and can then be seen on plain radiographs (Figure 7.7). Asymmetrical damage and swelling of the brain may cause deviation of the midline structures, as shown by the calcified

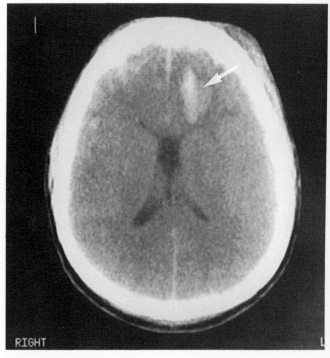

Fig. 7.6 CT brain scan showing left frontal haemorrhage due to trauma (→).

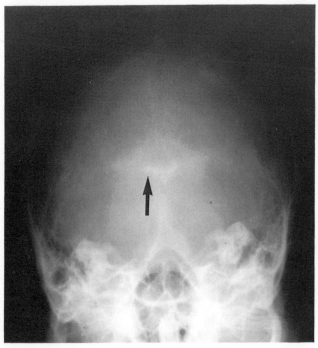

Fig. 7.7 AP radiograph of skull, showing calcified pineal displaced from the midline (→).

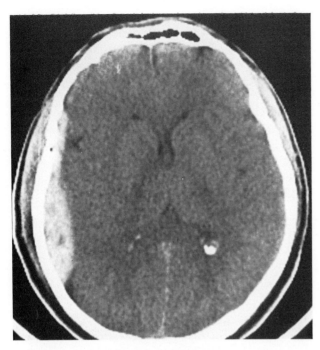

Fig. 7.8 Acute right subdural collection on CT scan.

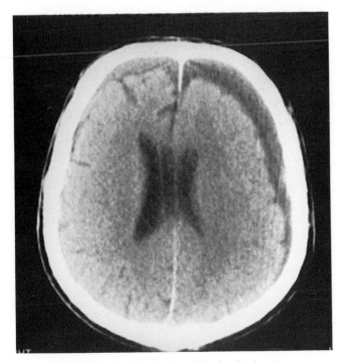

Fig. 7.9 Chronic low density subdural collections (hygromas) on CT scan.

pineal, if present, lying off-centre. Diffuse brain damage may show on CT as patchy oedema, with occasional micro-haemorrhages, often in the brain stem.

Extradural haematoma
This is a relatively uncommon injury, but may be rapidly progressive and associated with tears of meningeal arteries. Radiologically it is very similar to an acute subdural haematoma.

Acute subdural haematoma
This arises from tearing of veins crossing the subdural space. As with an extradural haematoma it is essentially a space occupying lesion.

Radiological appearances
1. Unilateral haematoma:
   (a) Plain radiographs. There may be displacement of the calcified pineal (visible on plain films in the midline in about 30% of adults) with possibly a skull fracture.
   (b) Computerized tomography. This shows the blood extremely reliably (Figure 7.8).
   (c) Angiography. The cortical vessels are shown separated from the inner table of the skull by the collection of blood.

Chronic subdural haematoma
This results if a small acute subdural collection is not drained. Increasing volume over time presents as a space occupying lesion.

Radiological appearances
1. The investigations for acute subdural haematoma as listed above show similar changes in chronic subdural haematoma (Figure 7.9).
2. Radionuclide scanning: the deviated vessels and hypervascular membrane around the collection may be shown.

Post-traumatic problems
These include localized or generalized atrophy, hydrocephalus, cysts or intracranial calcifications, and are all best seen by CT.

INTRACEREBRAL HAEMORRHAGE

A common form of 'stroke', intracerebral haemorrhage occurs usually in association with hypertension.

Radiological appearances

1. Computerized tomography: small haemorrhages, especially those in the brain stem, can be imaged by CT, in which the blood density is easily seen against the brain.

2. Plain radiographs: if the haematoma is large, causing significant displacement of brain tissue, it may also be detected on plain radiographs by shift of the (calcified) pineal.

3. Angiography: displacement of arteries and veins by the haemorrhage is shown.

Subependymal haemorrhage

This is common in premature infants and may readily be seen by CT or more usually by ultrasound via the fontanelle window (Figure 7.10).

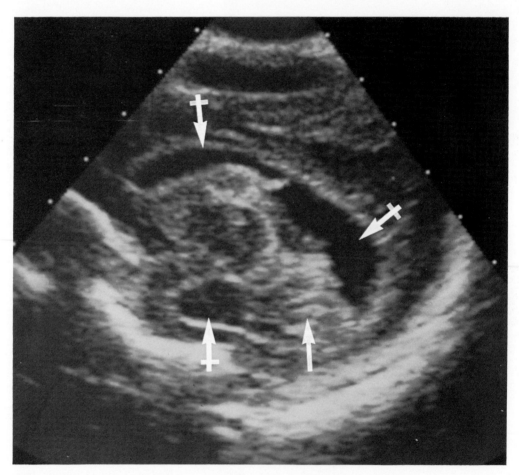

Fig. 7.10 Intraventricular blood clot in neonate, shown by ultrasound (→). Ventricle (↔).

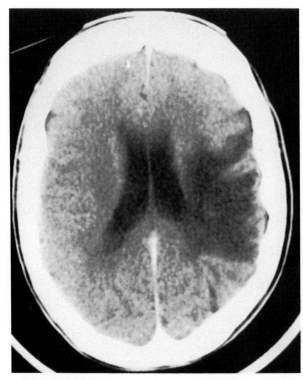

Fig. 7.11 CT scan showing left cerebral infarct.

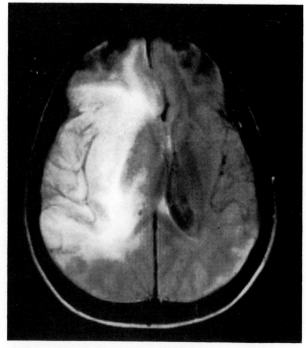

Fig. 7.12 Magnetic resonance scan showing right cerebral oedema, with displacement of ventricles in case of cerebral tumour. T2 weighted image (Philips Gyroscan, by courtesy of Philips Medical Systems Div, Eindhoven, The Netherlands).

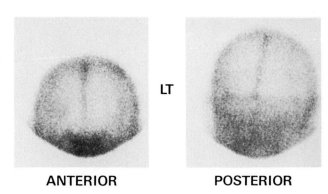

ANTERIOR   POSTERIOR   LT

RT LATERAL   LT LATERAL   A

CEREBRAL INFARCT
This also is a form of 'stroke'.

Radiological appearances
The same imaging tests as used in haemorrhage are appropriate, but with the following differences:

1. CT shows oedema only, with later scarring, unless there is secondary haemorrhage into the infarct (Figure 7.11).

2. MRI also shows oedema, unless secondary haemorrhage is present (Figure 7.12).

3. Angiography may show occluded vessels.

4. Radionuclide scanning may be useful in showing large infarcts, using pyrophosphate which accumulates in dying tissue (Figure 7.13). CT is, however, more sensitive and specific.

Fig. 7.13 Radionuclide brain scan, showing right middle cerebral infarct (→).

VASCULAR OCCLUSION OR STENOSIS

These may be intracranial or extracranial. The former usually produces infarcts related to the end-arteries blocked, and may be thrombotic or embolic from the heart or craniocervical vessels. Atheroma of the carotid or vertebral arteries may promote micro-embolization or, if stenosed, a degree of cerebral hypoxia — both being causes of transient ischaemic attacks (TIAs).

Radiological appearances

1. Ultrasound: vessel stenoses and flow abnormalities may be shown by B-mode ultrasound and Doppler studies (Fig. 7.14).

2. Angiography: the vessel lumen is displayed in detail (Fig. 7.15). The recent development of digital subtraction angiography has lead to much easier and more extensive utilization of angiography (Figure 7.16).

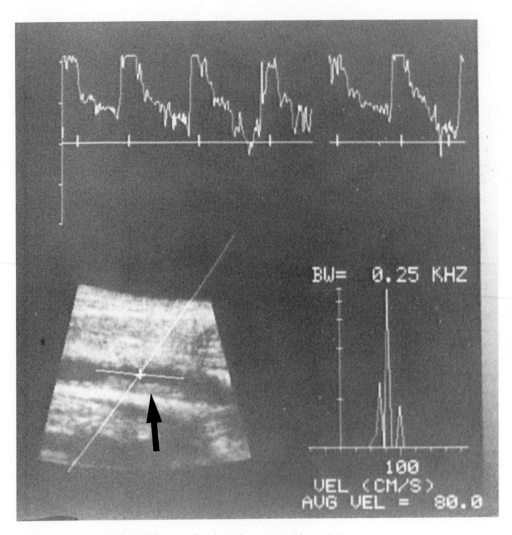

Fig. 7.14 Ultrasound of carotid artery showing atheromatous plaque (→) causing stenosis and the Doppler trace of the blood flow pattern.

TRANSIENT ISCHAEMIC ATTACKS

A suggested sequence of examinations for transient ischaemic attacks (TIAs) is shown in Diagnostic decision tree 6c, page 305.

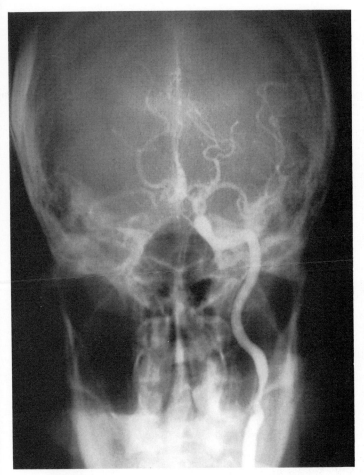

Fig. 7.15 AP projection of selective left carotid angiogram, showing stenosis at the origin of the internal carotid artery, occlusion of the external carotid, and cross-flow in the circle of Willis.

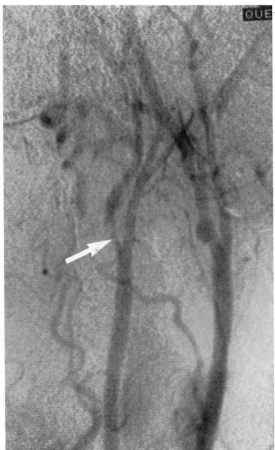

Fig. 7.16 Internal carotid artery stenosis demonstrated by intravenous digital subtraction angiography (→).

SUBARACHNOID HAEMORRHAGE (SAH)

This occasionally accompanies intracerebral bleeding but is usually due to rupture of either a congenital (berry) aneurysm or of an arteriovenous malformation (AVM).

Radiological appearances

1. Computerized tomography: the subarachnoid blood and any intracerebral haematoma or AVM is shown, but a small berry aneurysm can be missed.

2. Angiography: the size, shape, position and number of aneurysms are shown in great detail (Figure 7.17), as are the feeding and draining vessels of AVM. This information is essential in surgical intervention. Interventional radiology is also now playing a part in the treatment of intracranial lesions, especially by the transvascular obliteration of AVM and arteriovenous fistulas by artifical emboli.

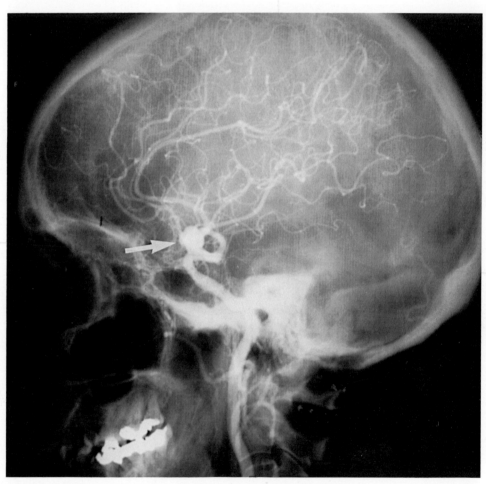

Fig. 7.17 Selective carotid angiogram showing an intracranial berry aneurysm (→).

NEOPLASMS

Neoplastic involvement of the brain may be due to either primary or secondary tumours, which usually present with either localized dysfunctional problems such as epilepsy, or raised intracranial pressure.

Neoplasms are best studied by CT, angiography and MRI but plain radiographs may show evidence of their presence.

Radiological appearance

1. Plain radiographs. There may be:
   (a) Displacement of a calcified pineal.
   (b) Sclerosis and thickening or rarefaction of the overlying skull bones.
   (c) An increase in the size and number of vascular markings on the skull in the region of the tumour.
   (d) Calcification in the mass (rarely).
   (e) Evidence of increased intracranial pressure (Figure 7.18) as indicated by the following: opening up of cranial suture lines; a generalized thinning of skull bones to give a copper-beaten appearance to the skull — this appearance should be discounted in infants; erosion of the posterior clinoid processes and dorsum sellae of the pituitary fossa; ballooning of the pituitary fossa and depression of its floor; erosion of the tip of the petrous temporal bone and widening of the internal auditory canal with some acoustic nerve tumours.

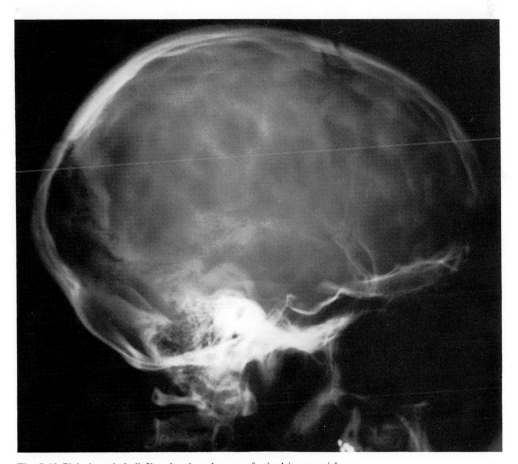

Fig. 7.18 Plain lateral skull film showing changes of raised intracranial pressure, i.e. 'copper-beaten' appearance and enlarged pituitary fossa.

2. Computerized tomography: this is a highly sensitive and specific investigation. Often no other test (except perhaps biopsy) is necessary. The relevant CT signs are the presence of a mass of abnormal density, shift of brain tissue, oedema and hypervascularity (Figure 7.19).

3. Angiography: if it is necessary to delineate feeding vessels or, in an AVM, the draining vessels this investigation does it well (Figure 7.20). There is usually evidence of pituitary lesions on plain radiographs but they are also best studied by CT (see 'Endocrine system',

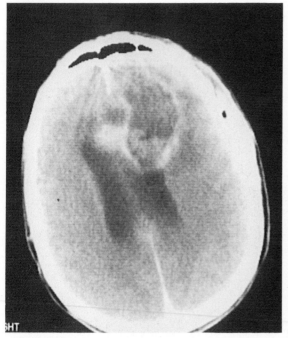

Fig. 7.19 Contrast enhanced CT scan showing frontal tumour.

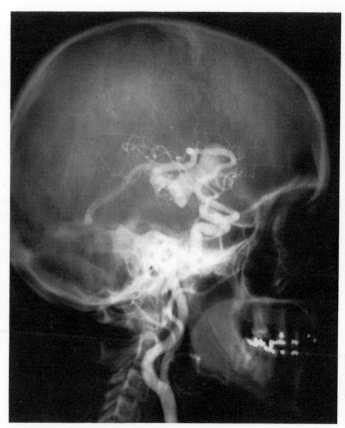

A

Fig. 7.20 Selective carotid angiograms of:
(A) arterio-venous malformation;
(B) hypervascular tumour (→).

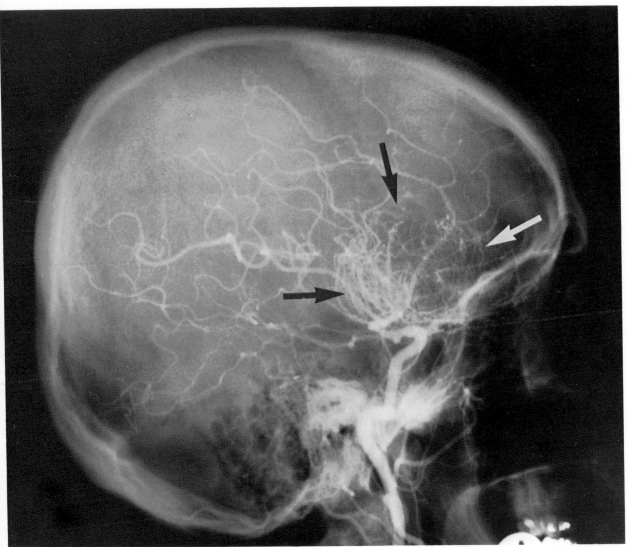

B

page 249). Magnetic resonance imaging
promises to be even more useful than CT in
neurological investigation, but ultrasound and
radionuclide scanning are of limited value
(Figure 7.21).

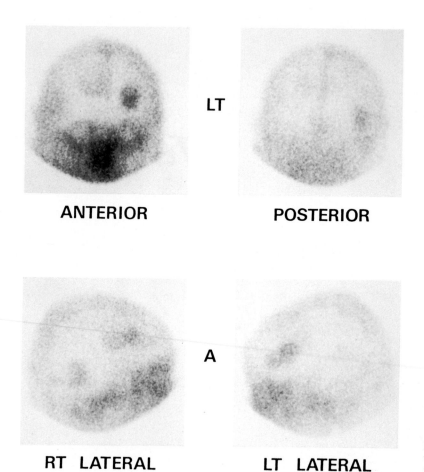

Fig. 7.21 Radionuclide brain scan with multiple tumour metastases from breast carcinoma.

INFLAMMATORY LESIONS

Abscess

This is often associated with infections of the paranasal or mastoid air cells, or with trauma. Abscesses may present in tumour-like fashion. Imaging investigations are similar to those for a tumour.

Radiological appearances

1. Computerized tomography: a peripheral hypervascular ring around the lesion is characteristic but not totally pathognomonic of an abscess (Figure 7.22).

2. Radionuclide scan: this is a highly sensitive but not very specific test.

Meningitis

Meningeal infections or infiltrations are not generally amenable to imaging tests although secondary hydrocephalus (page 231) is frequent.

Encephalitis

By virtue of the associated oedema and vascularity, encephalitis is well demonstrated by imaging.

Radiological appearances

1. Computerized tomography: oedema, tissue displacement, and vascularity are shown.

2. Radionuclide scan: the affected areas are 'hot'.

3. Magnetic resonance imaging: this shows oedema and tissue displacement.

The differentiation of encephalitis from tumour, abscess, infarct or demyelinating disease may be difficult in the acute state.

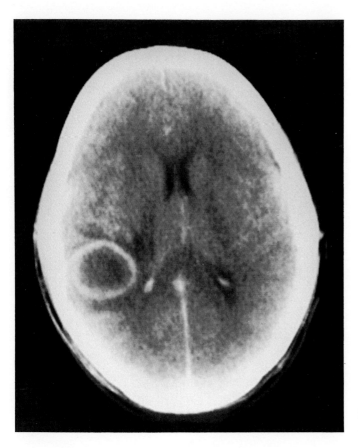

Fig. 7.22 Contrast enhanced CT scan of right parietal abscess.

DEMYELINATING DISEASES

As a group these have been difficult to diagnose, except by exclusion, but newer imaging modalities are helpful in both localizing and following the disease processes.

Radiological appearances

1. Computerized tomography: in the acute phase this demonstrates patchy loss of density, due to areas of oedema of white matter with spotty vascularity and little if any mass effect. As the lesion regresses there may be almost complete resolution of all these changes.

2. Magnetic resonance imaging: this is highly sensitive in showing demyelination and will probably become the investigation of choice (Figure 7.23).

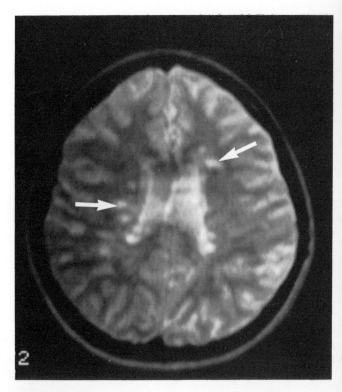

Fig. 7.23 Magnetic resonance scan (T2 weighted image) showing demyelinating lesions in multiple sclerosis (→) (Fonar MRI, by courtesy of Professor W Hanafee).

CEREBRAL ATROPHY

While this may be due to congenital abnormalities such as Alzheimer's disease, it is more commonly associated with age, possibly coupled with cerebro-vascular insufficiency.

Radiological appearances

1. Computerized tomography: ventricular dilatation and cortical atrophy with sulcal widening is shown (Figure 7.24).

2. Magnetic resonance imaging: this shows similar features to CT.

3. Pneumoencephalography: ventricular dilatation and cortical atrophy are shown but this examination has now been replaced by CT.

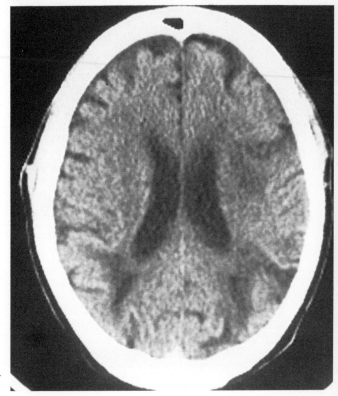

Fig. 7.24 Cortical gyral atrophy demonstrated by CT.

HYDROCEPHALUS

Ventricular dilatation occurs in association with cerebral atrophy but is most common and severe when associated with abnormalities of cerebrospinal fluid production, transit and reabsorption, and may occur at any age.

Radiological appearances

1. Ultrasound: hydrocephalus may be seen in the fetus by ultrasound, the ventricles and often the whole head being larger than normal (Figure 7.25). Intra-uterine surgery with shunting may have the potential to at least reduce the progress of this neuro-crippling lesion. After birth the hydrocephalic state is best studied by ultrasound up to 2–3 years of age.

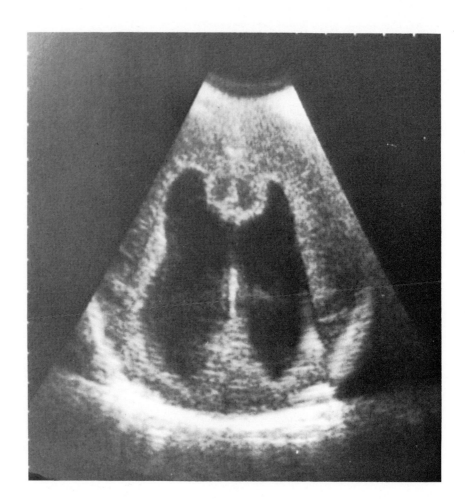

Fig. 7.25 Ultrasound of hydrocephalus in a neonate.

2. Computerized tomography: this is a valuable examination at any age (Figure 7.26). Pathological masses, obstructing the cerebrospinal fluid flow through and from the ventricles, can usually be seen by ultrasound in infants or by CT, which may also indicate the level of block by comparative ventricular sizes.

3. Nuclear medicine: communicating hydrocephalus, with obstruction to the flow of cerebrospinal fluid over the cortex or failure of absorption in the arachnoid villi (often because of previous subarachnoid bleeding or infection), is difficult to differentiate in some cases. It may require nuclear medicine cerebrospinal fluid studies, showing abnormal transit and slow absorption.

The effectiveness of shunts (ventriculo-atrial or ventriculo-peritoneal) is readily monitored by ultrasound in infants or CT in adults, by comparison of ventricular sizes over a period of time.

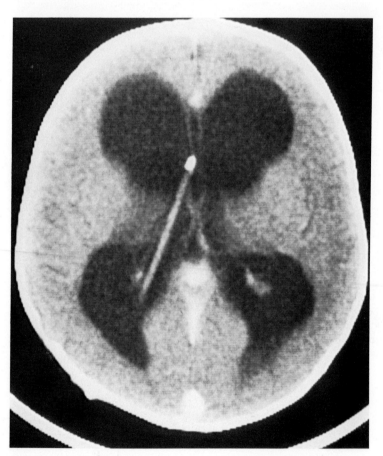

Fig. 7.26 Hydrocephalus subsequent to birth trauma, shown by CT. Part of ventriculo-peritoneal shunt is shown.

HEADACHE
Headache is a common presenting symptom of brain pathology. A suggested sequence of imaging investigations is shown in Diagnostic decision tree 6a, page 304.

The spinal cord

METHODS OF INVESTIGATION

While the tissues of the spinal cord are similar to those of the brain, the frequency of specific pathologies is quite different and the investigations are of different importance.

Plain radiographs
These are of major importance, especially in the assessment of lesions secondary to trauma or spinal degeneration. Antero-posterior, lateral and oblique films are the minimal requirement except in unstable fractures when difficulty in moving the patient may limit the examination.

The integrity of the vertebrae and discs is usually assessable.

Computerized tomography
This is the outstanding non-invasive examination for the bony structures and, to a lesser extent, the cord and its surrounding soft tissues. Spinal stenosis, disc lesions, haematomas and tumours are usually readily seen.

Magnetic resonance imaging
Magnetic resonance imaging shows great promise as a non-invasive investigation, potentially surpassing CT in soft tissue analysis (Figure 7.27).

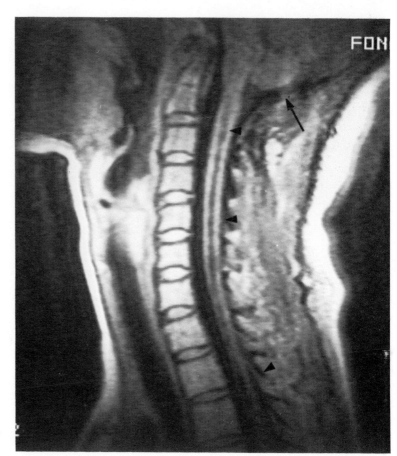

Fig. 7.27 Magnetic resonance image of cervical region showing mild hydromyelia (▶) (Fonar MRI, by courtesy of Professor W Hanafee).

Myelography
This is performed by subarachnoid instillation of radio-opaque contrast medium by lumbar puncture (Figure 7.28). It is a sensitive method of showing intrathecal lesions and, by displacement of the theca, the presence of significant extrathecal masses, particularly tumours and disc protrusions.

Radionuclide scan
This has little to offer except in the demonstration of active pathological processes in adjacent bone structures.

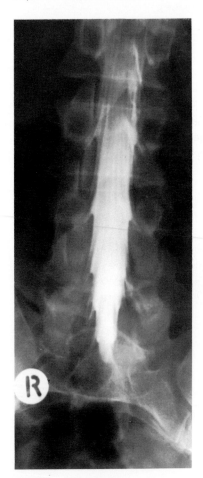

Fig. 7.28 Normal lumbar myelogram, AP projection.

LESIONS OF THE SPINAL CORD

CONGENITAL LESIONS
Developmental anomalies are relatively common, ranging from mild (usually inconsequential) spina bifida occulta, through meningocoele and hydrocephalus, to gross deformities such as anencephaly. Lesions are commonly multiple.

Hydrocephaly
Investigation is as indicated (see page 231), but it may be associated with other lesions such as toxoplasmosis (usually an intra-uterine infection) or more commonly with a degree of rachischisis, cord tethering and Arnold–Chiari malformation.

Anencephaly
This defect is incompatible with life and may be diagnosed antenatally by ultrasound or radiography (Figure 7.29).

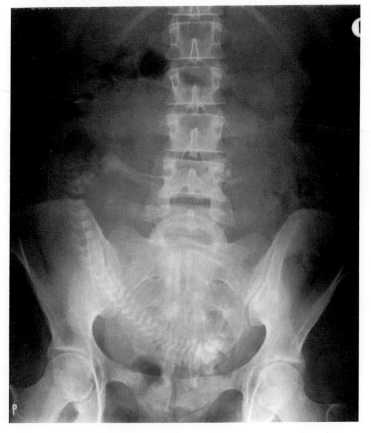

Fig. 7.29 Plain radiograph of pregnant abdomen, at 33 weeks gestation. Absence of visible skull vault indicates anencephaly.

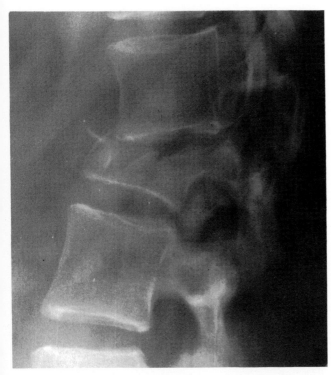

Fig. 7.30 Lateral radiograph of lumbar spine showing wedge fracture of vertebral body.

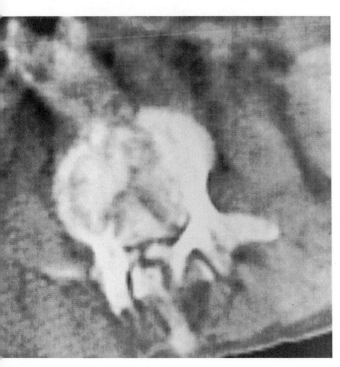

Fig. 7.31 CT scan of vertebra in Figure 7.30, showing the gross degree of destruction and displacement of fragments not readily appreciable on plain films.

Spinal defects

These range from spina bifida occulta to meningo-myelocele, usually involving the lumbar spine. Antenatal diagnosis is important in the more severe defects and may be made by ultrasound, even in some cases as early as 16 weeks gestation.

Postnatally, clinical studies and plain films provide most of the necessary data, particularly of the bony spine. Additional information on the soft tissues may be acquired by CT, which is especially valuable around the base of the skull, and myelography using either positive contrast medium or gas to show the thecal and cord anatomy in detail.

TRAUMA

The neurological problems associated with the cord are generally due to pressure from a haematoma, oedema or bone, consequent on fractures or dislocations of the spine, or from prolapse of intervertebral disc material.

Radiological appearances

1. Plain radiographs: these provide much information on bony damage and are essential (Figure 7.30).

2. Computerized tomography: this may be necessary to show occult fractures, the detailed disposition of the bone fragments, and soft tissue masses such as an extradural haematoma (Figure 7.31).

3. Myelography: this may be required to show the integrity or otherwise of the spinal cord and nerve roots.

4. Magnetic resonance imaging: this examination promises to provide much valuable non-invasive information.

INTERVERTEBRAL DISC LESIONS

These are usually associated with trauma or degeneration, involving principally the cervical and lumbar spine. Investigation is the same as for trauma with the possible addition of epidural venography as an indirect method of showing the presence of space-occupying lesion(s) in the extrathecal part of the spinal canal.

Myelography will show indentation of the theca by protruded disc material (Figure 7.32).

Computerized tomography is used preferentially (Figure 7.33).

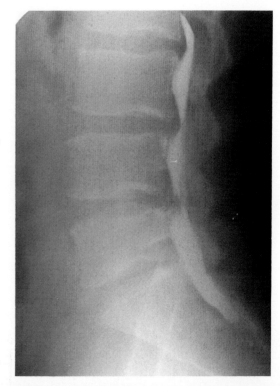

Fig. 7.32 Lateral radiograph of lumbar myelogram showing backward displacement of theca by a herniated disc.

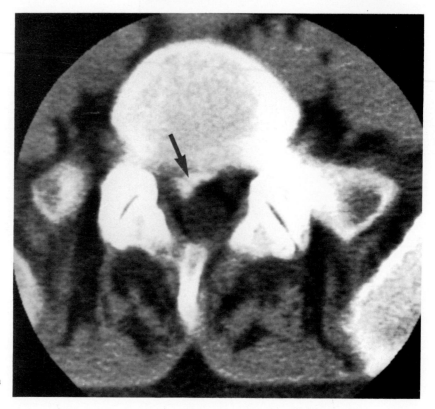

Fig. 7.33 Calcified herniated lumbar disc fragment (→) shown on CT scan.

INFLAMMATORY LESIONS

These relatively uncommon lesions include extrathecal infections, usually abscesses, often arising from discitis or spinal osteomyelitis and behaving like an extradural space-occupying lesion — with appropriate investigation as above.

Meningitis

Inflammatory conditions of the theca are not generally amenable to imaging.

Myelitis

This is to a large extent a diagnosis of exclusion, but may show as a swollen cord on myelography, CT and possibly in the future specifically on MRI.

DEGENERATIVE DISEASES OF THE CORD

These are not usefully imaged. Degeneration of the spine itself, however, is important as the secondary effects, such as disc narrowing and protrusion and posterior joint osteophytosis, commonly lead to pressure damage to either the cord or the nerve roots (Figure 7.34).

Investigation is the same as for trauma and disc disease.

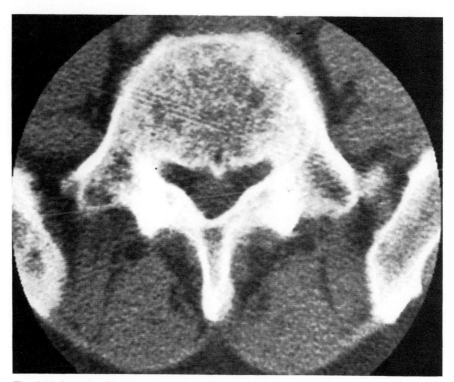

Fig. 7.34 Stenosis of lumbar spinal canal, demonstrated by CT.

NEOPLASMS

Tumours may be benign or malignant, intrathecal or extrathecal, primary or secondary. By far the most common is secondary, malignant and extrathecal, often involving vertebrae and also the central nervous system by pressure from the mass or vertebral collapse. Investigation is usually by the same sequence of tests as for trauma or disc lesions.

Radiological appearances

1. Plain radiographs: these may show destruction of bone or pathological calcification.

2. Computerized tomography: this is the most sensitive examination and may show bone destruction, a soft tissue mass and perhaps calcification.

3. Myelography: an intrathecal mass, a block of the subarachnoid space, or indentation by an extrathecal mass may be shown (Figure 7.35).

4. Angiography: this is useful only if a vascular lesion, such as an AVM is suspected.

5. Radionuclide scan: active and otherwise often occult lesions in the spine may be demonstrated.

The peripheral nerves are generally not amenable to imaging. Neurofibromatosis, however, may present on images by virtue of soft tissue masses or bone defects (tibia and fibula, ribs, posterior wall of orbit) due to pressure from the tumours, and may be associated with acoustic nerve neuromas.

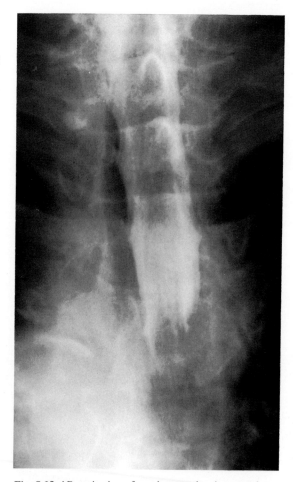

Fig. 7.35 AP projection of myelogram showing complete extradural block in upper thoracic region due to tumour.

SCIATICA

Sciatica is a common presenting symptom of pathology involving the lower cord and corda equina. A suggested sequence of imaging investigations for this symptom is shown in Diagnostic decision tree 6b, page 305.

The eye

Intrabulbar lesions are generally visible to external or ophthalmoscopic view, but imaging is useful in trauma when foreign bodies may be localized by radiography (if radio-opaque) or occasionally by CT or ultrasound.

Retrobulbar lesions, often leading to exophthalmos, are best investigated by high resolution CT scanning (Figure 7.36), which clearly demonstrates the muscle cone, the nerve and occasionally the vessels. Angiography may rarely be necessary in angiomatous lesions.

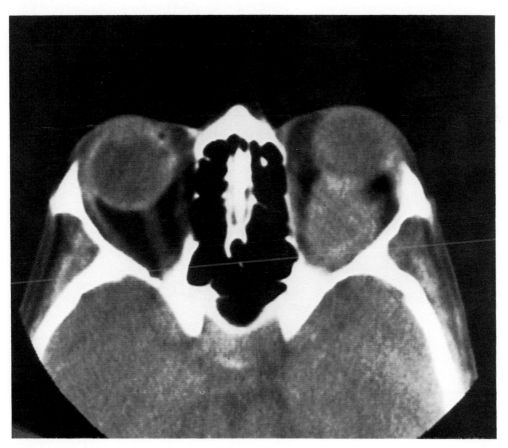

Fig. 7.36 CT scan of orbits, showing a large left retrobular mass.

8 The Endocrine System

The development of sophisticated biochemical methods of hormone assay have not only dramatically improved the detection and diagnosis of endocrine disease, but have required much more accurate imaging techniques for lesion localization and characterization.

The thyroid

Diseases of the thyroid are relatively common, presenting principally with hyperthyroidism, hypothyroidism, or a mass in the neck.

HYPERTHYROIDISM OR THYROTOXICOSIS
This is due to overproduction of thyroid hormones and is diagnosed biochemically.

Radiological appearances
1. Plain radiographs: displacement and/or narrowing of the trachea may occur (Figure 8.1).
2. Nuclear medicine: radioactive iodine (^{131}I or ^{123}I) uptake studies determine the rate of trapping and organification of iodine. They are mostly used as a factor in prescribing the dose for ^{131}I therapy.
3. Radionuclide scan: using I-131, I-123 or, most commonly, Tc-99m as pertechnetate the thyroid can be scanned. The scan shows the shape, size and position of active thyroid tissue. In diffuse hyperplasia the whole gland is large and 'hot' (Figure 8.2). Toxic nodules or adenomas will show as localized areas of high activity.

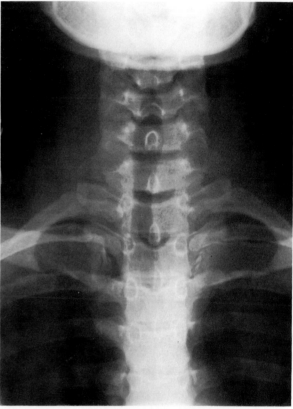

Fig. 8.1 Radiograph of thoracic inlet, showing displacement and narrowing of trachea by enlarged lobe of thyroid.

HYPOTHYROIDISM
While usually primary or due to thyroiditis, it may also occur with iodine deficiency, dyshormonogenesis, or previous therapy. Congenital hypoplasia, aplasia, or lack of thyroid stimulating hormone may also be causative.

Radiological appearances
1. Nuclear medicine: ^{131}I uptake with perchlorate discharge may quantify trapping abnormalities, but imaging tests are of little value.

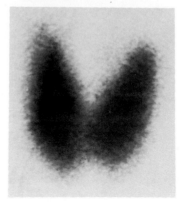

Fig. 8.2 Radionuclide scan of diffuse hyperplasia of thyroid.

2. Plain radiographs: secondary effects such as cretinism may be occasionally diagnosed on plain skeletal radiography showing delayed epiphyseal development with stippled calcification of the epiphyses.

NODULAR GOITRE

The most common benign mass is a non-toxic goitre with nodular gland enlargement.

Radiological appearances

1. Radionuclide scan: technesium-99m is used. The large gland shows patchy uptake indicating variable topical function (Figure 8.3).

2. Ultrasound: this will also show the presence of nodules and their consistency, which may be solid or cystic (Figure 8.4). Differentiation between benign and malignant solid masses is unreliable.

3. Plain radiographs: films of the neck and thoracic inlet may show retrosternal extension, calcification in nodules and deviation or compression of the trachea.

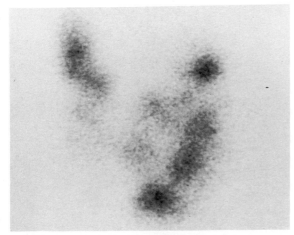

Fig. 8.3 Radionuclide scan of multinodular goitre.

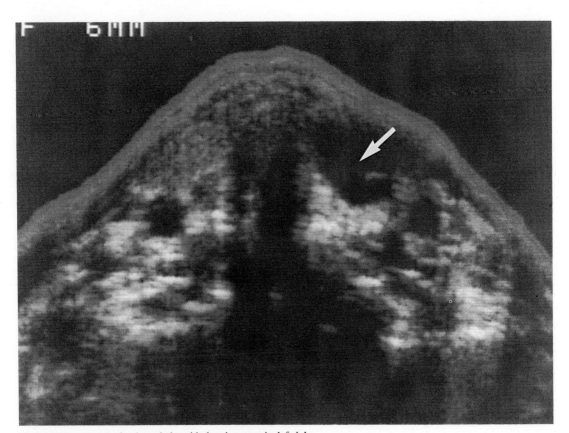

Fig. 8.4 Ultrasound of enlarged thyroid showing cyst in left lobe.

BENIGN ADENOMAS
Solitary or multiple adenomas may be hormonally active or inactive.

Radiological appearances
A radionuclide scan will show whether the adenoma is active, permitting rational therapy (Figure 8.5). It is virtually impossible to differentiate between benign and malignant solitary solid 'cold' nodules without biopsy or excision.

AUTO-IMMUNE THYROIDITIS
Clinical presentation includes thyroid swelling, often tender, with transient hyperthyroidism.

   A radionuclide thyroid scan will show patchy, low uptake of the radionuclide.

MALIGNANT TUMOURS
Malignancies of the thyroid are relatively uncommon and usually present as a mass.

Radiological appearances
   1. Radionuclide scan: the mass is cold (see Figure 8.5).
   2. Ultrasound: the mass is solid, sometimes with ill defined margins (Figure 8.6).
   3. Chest radiographs: these are used to check for metastases.

THYROID MASS
A suggested sequence of imaging examinations for a palpable thyroid mass is shown in Diagnostic decision tree 7, page 306.

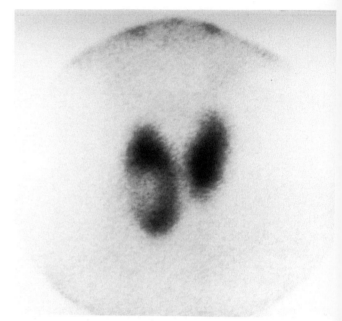

Fig. 8.5 Radionuclide thyroid scan showing solitary cold nodule in right lobe.

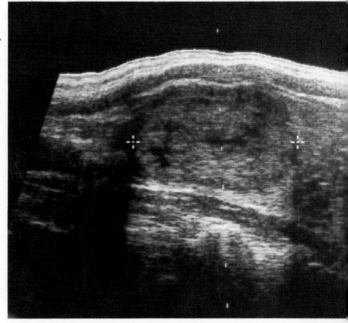

Fig. 8.6 Ultrasound of thyroid showing a cold nodule to be solid.

The parathyroids

The parathyroids are a set of four small glands normally lying in the neck. The only significant lesions are associated with hyposecretion or hypersecretion of parathormone.

HYPERPARATHYROIDISM

This is due to primary hyperplasia, adenoma, or rarely carcinoma (see Chapter 6, page 210).

Radiological appearances

1. Ultrasound: the neck is examined to attempt to identify one or more enlarged parathyroids, usually on the posterior aspect of the thyroid.

2. Computerized tomography: this may also show enlarged parathyroid glands in the neck or upper mediastinum.

3. Percutaneous catheter sampling: examination of blood from the draining veins in the neck and upper mediastinum, may localize the site of hormone hyperproduction.

4. Plain radiographs: films of the skeleton may show subperiosteal bone resorption, especially in the phalanges (see Figure 6.73), and less commonly the cystic 'brown tumours' of Von Recklinghausen's disease.

HYPOPARATHYROIDISM

This may be primary or secondary (usually following thyroid surgery). Imaging plays little part in its investigation, but plain radiographs may show calcification in soft tissue, especially the basal ganglia of the brain, and, in the congenital type, shortened metacarpals.

The adrenals

The majority of adrenal syndromes relate to hypersecretion or hyposecretion of medullary or cortical hormones and are primarily clinical and biochemical diagnoses.

ATROPHY
This is usually associated with previous tuberculosis, infarction, auto-immune disease or medical therapy, and is not amenable to imaging.

HYPERTROPHY
This is usually bilateral with hyperhormonogenesis.

Radiological appearances
1. Computerized tomography: the size, shape and position of the adrenals are well shown.

2. Radionuclide scan: iodocholesterol compounds which are concentrated in the adrenal are used and may provide differential adrenal activity estimations.

ADENOMA
Adrenal adenomas usually present due to hormonal hypersecretion.

Radiological appearances
1. Computerized tomography (Figure 8.7).
2. Venous blood sampling for hormone analysis by selective percutaneous catherization.
3. Angiography: this may show a pathological circulation if it is present in the adenoma.

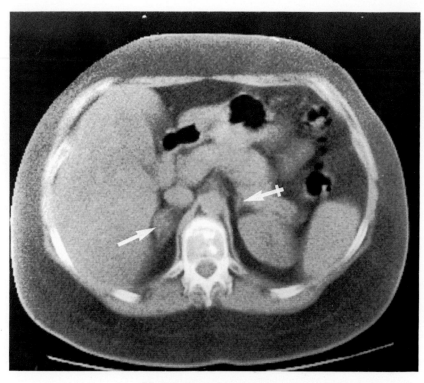

Fig. 8.7 CT of abdomen demonstrating both adrenal glands. Normal left adrenal (↦); right adrenal adenoma (→).

NEUROBLASTOMA
This tumour occurs in infancy.

Radiological appearances

1. Ultrasound: the solid mass displacing the kidney and liver is displayed.

2. Computerized tomography: this produces the same signs as ultrasound (Figure 8.8).

3. Intravenous pyelography: the displacement of the kidney is shown and helps to differentiate a neuroblastoma from a Wilm's tumour of the kidney.

4. Skeletal radiographs: these are used to detect metastases.

5. Angiography: pathological vessels in the tumour are shown but significant additional information is rarely produced.

CARCINOMA
Malignant tumours of the adrenal are often non-active hormonally and are investigated as for neuroblastoma, with emphasis on CT. Adenomas or carcinomas with high hormone production are also investigated as for neuroblastoma, but in addition percutaneous catheter venous sampling and hormone assay may help to localize active lesions, especially in phaeochromocytomas, which are frequently multiple and ectopic in situation.

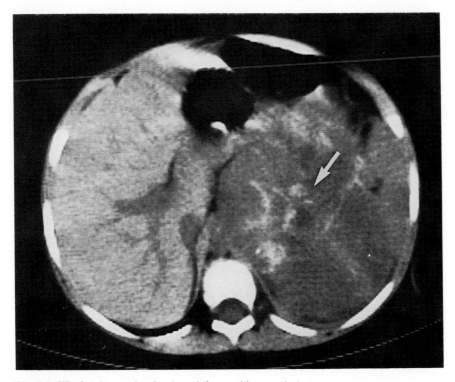

Fig. 8.8 CT of abdomen showing large left neuroblastoma (→).

Pancreas — endocrine

Most of the appropriate imaging tests for pancreas have been noted in the gastrointestinal section (Chapter 4). Diabetes may be associated with a pancreatic tumour, atrophy or chronic pancreatitis, but is of itself rarely an indication for imaging tests.

HYPERFUNCTION OF ISLET CELLS
This is associated with islet cell tumours either benign or malignant, or, on occasion, with hyperplasia.

Radiological appearances
1. Computerized tomography: this is reasonably sensitive in showing tumours and is the test of choice (Figure 8.9).
2. Ultrasound: this is less sensitive than C T, especially for lesions in the pancreatic tail.
3. Angiography: a mass with pathological vessels may be shown.
4. Percutaneous transhepatic portal vein catheterization: with blood sampling along the splenic vein and hormone assay, this may help to localize an otherwise occult tumour.

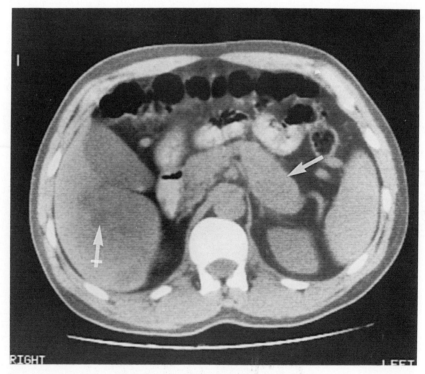

Fig. 8.9 CT of pancreas showing mass in the tail of the gland (→).
This proved to be a malignant islet cell tumour with liver metastases (↔).

Pituitary

The diagnosis of pituitary pathology is usually biochemically based, although occasionally the mass effect of a tumour will cause presenting symptoms such as bitemporal hemianopia. Specific hormonal dysfunctions may be due to small or large tumours, atrophy, or overdriving by stimulating hormones.

Radiological appearances

1. Plain radiographs: films of the skull with localized views of the pituitary fossa. In most cases of small masses the appearances are normal, but large pituitary masses or an 'empty sella' (see page 250) may cause a large fossa, which may be symmetrical or asymmetrical (Figure 8.10). A suprasellar mass, such as a craniopharyngioma, may show erosion of the top of the posterior clinoid processes. Tomography may also help to delineate the sellar floor which may be thinned and depressed.

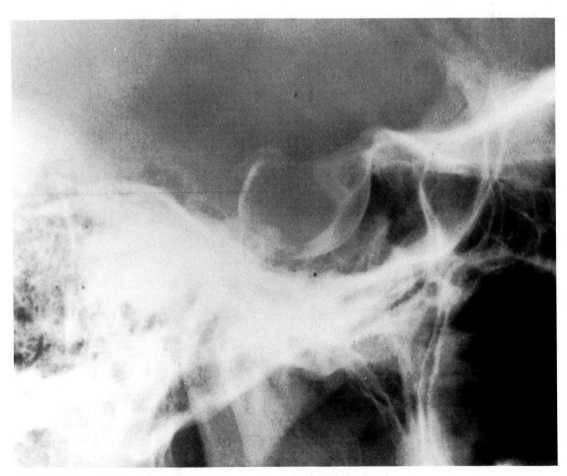

Fig. 8.10 Enlarged pituitary fossa shown on lateral radiograph of skull (detail).

2. Computerized tomography: this is the preferred examination using thin sections (about 2 mm thick) through the fossa both before and after intravenous instillation of urographic contrast medium, and with sagittal and coronal reconstruction. The urographic contrast medium circulating in the capillaries enhances the difference in the radiographic density of tissue and this produces better definition of tissues on the scan. Large masses will show destruction of the sellar bony margins, with or without extension into the paranasal air sinuses, displacement of the cavernous sinus, and sometimes upward bulging of, or extension through, the diaphragma sellae (Figure 8.11). Empty sella shows virtually only cerebrospinal fluid in the fossa with a small or no residual gland.

3. Angiography: this is used only in the differentiation between an intrasellar tumour and an aneurysm in that region.

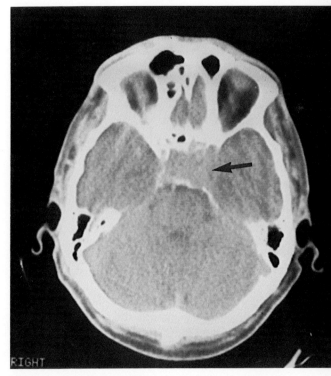

Fig. 8.11 CT of base of skull showing expansion and destruction of pituitary fossa.

9 Urinary Tract

METHODS OF INVESTIGATION

Plain radiographs

Plain films of the urinary tract should be made before any contrast examination, since areas of calcification and opaque calculi may be invisible when surrounded by contrast medium.

The plain film reveals any abnormality in the size, shape or position of the kidneys, and any opacities such as opaque calculi or calcification in the tract. Kidney size varies with the height of the individual but in adults averages between 12 and 15 cm in length. A normal kidney usually extends in length over a distance equal to $3\frac{1}{2}$ lumbar vertebrae, including the intervening discs, and this may be used as a rough measure of kidney size.

Intravenous pyelography

Contrast medium injected intravenously is rapidly excreted by the kidneys and the first film of the kidneys should be made five minutes after the injection. The ureters are then compressed by a tight band around the lower abdomen to allow good filling of the pelvis and calyces with contrast medium and further films made of the pyelograms at five minute intervals until the pelvis and calyces have been well visualized (Figure 9.1). The compression of the ureters is then released which allows the ureters and bladder to fill. After films of these structures have been made the patient is asked to void and a post-micturition film of the urinary tract is made (Figure 9.2).

Normal appearances:

1. The calyces in the two kidneys are roughly symmetrically placed and are arranged in upper, middle and lower groups (see Figure 9.1). They have a sharply defined concave outer end where the renal pyramids project into the calyces.

2. The pelvis is cone shaped and tapers evenly towards the upper end of the ureter.

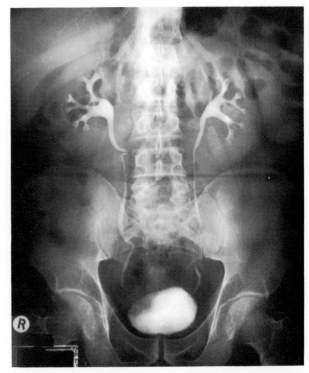

Fig. 9.1 Normal intravenous pyelogram.

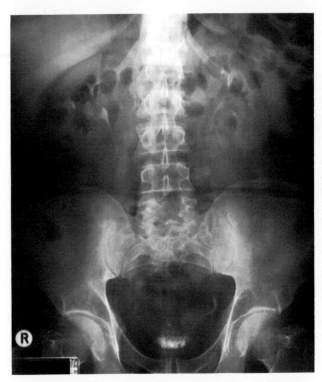

Fig. 9.2 Post-micturition film of normal intravenous pyelogram.

3. A line drawn through the tips of the outer pyramids of the kidney is called the interpapillary line and runs roughly parallel to the renal outline (Figure 9.3). The distance between this line and the kidney margin, usually about 1 cm, represents the thickness of the renal substance, which is usually slightly thicker at the upper and lower poles.

4. When the contrast medium enters the kidney it is distributed in the capillaries and renal tubules before excretion into the collecting system; as a result the kidney becomes more radio-opaque. This is termed a nephrogram or nephrogram stage of the intravenous pyelogram.

5. The ureters may show some peristaltic waves but otherwise the walls are parallel. The ureters cross the tips of the lumbar transverse processes and on entering the skeletal pelvis run in a curved course convex laterally to reach the bladder.

6. The bladder is smooth in outline and round except when there is pressure from the uterus which produces a smooth depression on the upper surface. The film made after micturition should show the bladder empty.

Retrograde pyelography
Ureteric catheters are placed in position through a cystoscope and contrast medium is injected to fill the pelvi-calyceal systems and ureters. Since modern intravenous contrast media produce such good visualization of the pelvi-calyceal structures, retrograde pyelography is now rarely performed, except perhaps when there is a non-functioning kidney present on an intravenous pyelogram.

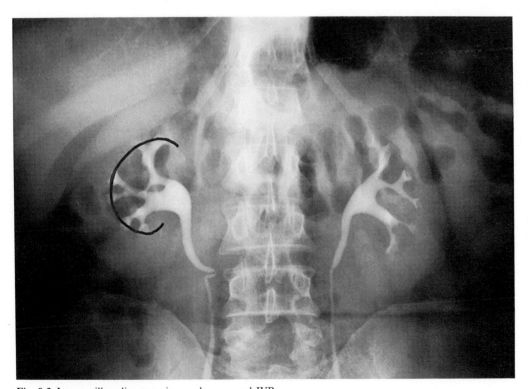

Fig. 9.3 Interpapillary line superimposed on normal IVP.

Cystography

The bladder is filled per urethra with contrast medium which may fill diverticula and outline tumours. Films made during straining or micturition may reveal vesico-ureteric reflux. Films made during micturition (cysto-urethrography) will show the urethra outlined by the contrast medium (Figure 9.4). This is the only method by which urethral valves are demonstrated.

Urethrography

The urethra is filled with contrast medium in a retrograde fashion. It is used to demonstrate strictures, ruptures, false passages and prostatic size. Micturating cysto-urethrography is sometimes a better method of examination.

Renal arteriography

A catheter is inserted percutaneously into the femoral artery in the groin and passed up into the aorta and into a renal artery. Contrast medium is then injected and outlines the renal circulation (Figure 9.5). This examination was previously used to differentiate between a cyst and a tumour but this role has now been taken over by ultrasound scanning and CT, although it is still of value in determining the degree of vascularity of, and renal vein involvement by, a tumour. Digital subtraction angiography produces good studies of the renal arteries by intravenous injection of contrast medium, but intrarenal detail is generally not adequate for showing very small vessels when selective angiography using either film or digital recording is required.

Cyst puncture

A long needle is passed percutaneously under x-ray or ultrasound control into the kidney to enter a cyst into which contrast medium is injected, and from which fluid is aspirated for cytological analysis.

Ultrasound

Ultrasound is a simple, rapid, non-traumatic method of investigating the renal tract. Normal ureters cannot be seen but the bladder and its

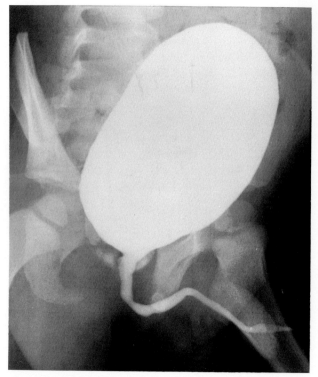

Fig. 9.4 Normal bladder and urethra shown by micturating cysto-urethrogram.

wall thickness is well shown since the fluid content is an excellent acoustic window.

Normal appearances:
1. The kidney parenchyma is relatively sonolucent although the columns of Bertin may show clearly (Figure 9.6).
2. The pelvis and calyces are obscured by intrarenal fat unless they are sufficiently dilated and then appear as sonolucent fluid-filled structures.
3. Renal arteries and veins are usually seen.
4. The bladder is best seen when full, when the inner aspect and wall thickness are clearly shown.

Computerized tomography

The size, shape and position of the kidneys, ureters and bladder are well shown on cross-sectional images or in coronal and sagittal reconstructions. The function may also be

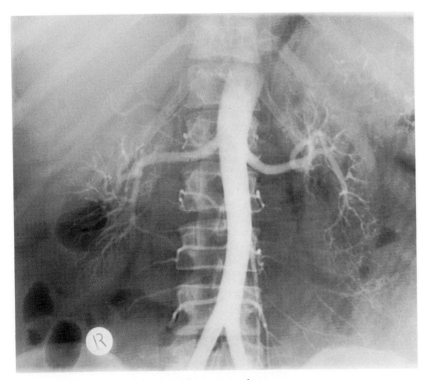

Fig. 9.5 Normal renal arteries shown by aortography.

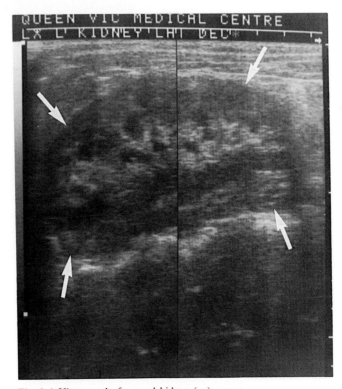

Fig. 9.6 Ultrasound of normal kidney (→).

assessed by the intravenous injection of urographic contrast medium. Rapid segmental scanning of an intravenous contrast bolus injection is now being used to determine the relative renal and segmental vascularity.

Radionuclide scan

Anatomical detail is poor because of the limited spatial resolution of radionuclide scanning, but quantitative physiological studies are of major value. Injection of inulin analogues (e.g. DTPA–Te-99m) or actively excreted materials (such as iodine labelled ortho-iodo-hippuric acid) with computer collection and analysis of data over 30 minutes or more demonstrates initial relative renal blood flow, concentration and excretion. Blood samples will quantitate the glomerular filtration rate (GFR). Urine transit to bladder, ureteric reflux and bladder emptying can also be quantified.

LESIONS OF THE KIDNEYS AND URETERS

CONGENITAL ABNORMALITIES

Renal agenesis

Congenital absence of one kidney is uncommon but when it exists the single kidney present is markedly hypertrophied but is otherwise normal in appearance. Computerized tomography and angiography may be required to be sure that only one kidney is present, as opposed to only one kidney functioning.

Renal hypoplasia

The kidney is small but is otherwise normal in appearance. The other kidney is hypertrophied.

Unilateral renal ischaemia may simulate renal hypoplasia; however, the latter has a small but normal renal artery, shown by angiography, in contrast to the narrowing seen in ischaemia.

Renal ectopia and malrotation

The kidneys originate within the skeletal pelvis and during development they ascend to the usual position in the abdomen. A kidney may fail to ascend — pelvic kidney — or its ascent may be arrested anywhere between the pelvis and the usual kidney position (Figure 9.7). Occasionally during ascent it may cross to the opposite side of the abdomen and may fuse with the kidney already there.

During its ascent the kidney rotates around its long axis so that the calyces which originally pointed medially now point laterally and the renal pelvis is now on the medial aspect of the kidney. A kidney may fail to rotate or may be incompletely rotated.

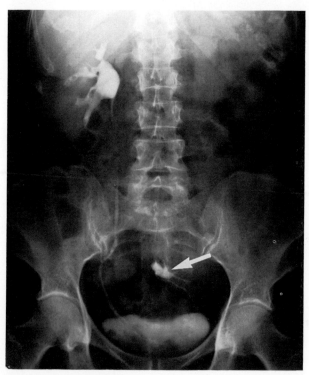

Fig. 9.7 Intravenous pyelogram showing left pelvic kidney.

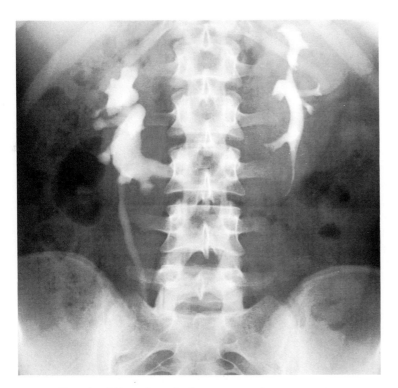

Fig. 9.8 Horseshoe kidney shown by intravenous pyelogram.

Horse-shoe kidney

The lower poles of the kidneys are united by a bridge of renal tissue. As a result the kidneys are unable to rotate and lie lower than usual in the abdomen. The lowest calyx on each side points medially instead of laterally (Figure 9.8).

Duplex kidney

Not uncommonly, a kidney may have two distinct pelvi-calyceal systems. This may be associated with a completely double ureter or the two ureters may fuse at any point between the renal pelvis and the bladder (Figure 9.9).

When they remain separate, the ureter from the upper pole system always enters the bladder below the ureter from the lower pole. It may also have an ectopic insertion into the urethra, uterus or vagina, and may be a cause of enuresis and recurrent urinary infection. A kidney with a double pelvi-calyceal system is bigger than the normal kidney on the opposite side.

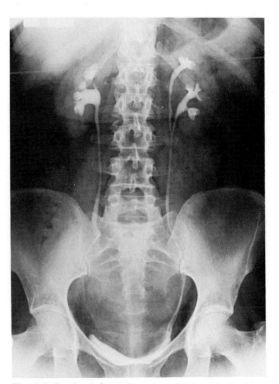

Fig. 9.9 Duplex left renal system at IVP, with double ureters extending to the bladder.

Ureterocoele

A ureterocoele is a congenital dilatation of the distal end of the ureter. In the cystogram phase of the pyelogram it is seen as a round dense area with a ring of radiolucency around it, towards the base of the bladder. The resulting 'cobra-head' appearance is diagnostic (Figure 9.10). Calculi may form in a ureterocoele.

Congenital hydronephrosis

The cause is uncertain but the condition is usually bilateral. The dilatation of the renal pelvis and calyces may be gross and associated with very poor function of the kidney, or it may only be moderate with reasonably good renal function.

Urethral valves

Congenital valves may occur in the posterior part of the male urethra and may cause marked obstruction with consequent severe dilatation of the bladder, ureters, renal pelves, and calyces. The abnormality is best shown in a voiding cysto-urethrogram (Figure 9.11).

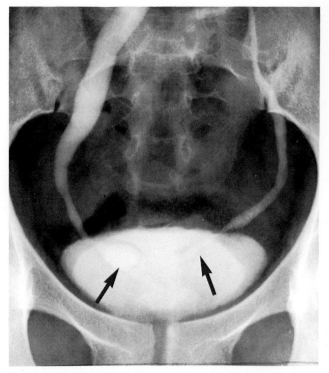

Fig. 9.10 Bladder at IVP, showing bilateral ureteroceles.

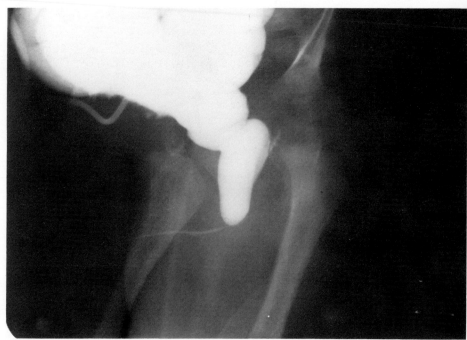

Fig. 9.11 Urethral valves causing obstruction, shown by micturating cysto-urethrogram.

MEDULLARY SPONGE KIDNEY (TUBULAR ECTASIA)

This is a condition in which there are large numbers of cysts in the medulla producing a spongy appearance. These cysts connect with the renal tubules which are irregular and dilated. The lesions may involve either or both kidneys in part or completely. In a very high percentage of cases calculi form in the dilated tubules.

Radiological appearances (Figure 9.12)

1. Smooth enlargement of the involved kidney.

2. Multiple small dense calculi in the medulla.

3. Fine irregular streaks of contrast medium radiating from the papilla into the medulla due to filling of dilated tubules during a pyelogram.

4. Widening of the calyces in the affected areas.

Medullary sponge kidney may be differentiated from other causes of nephrocalcinosis by the enlarged and widened calyces.

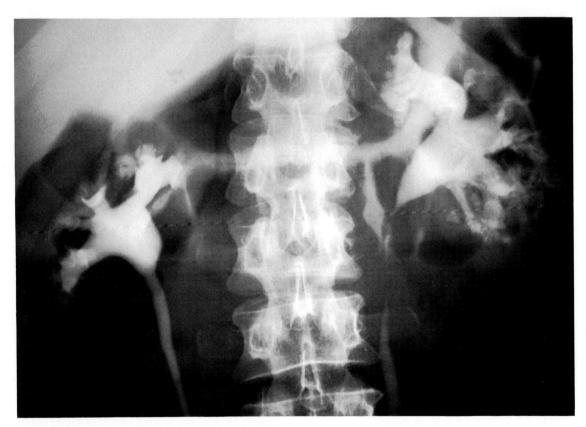

Fig. 9.12 Medullary sponge kidney (tubular ectasia) IVP showing dilated collecting ducts containing calculi.

RENAL TRAUMA

The most important function of radiology in cases of suspected renal trauma is to demonstrate a *normal*, functioning kidney on the opposite side.

Radiological appearances

1. Plain radiographs are often of little value because bowel gas shadows obscure the renal outlines and retroperitoneal structures. The following features may, however, be seen when the tear involves the capsule as well as the renal substance:

    (a) Loss of the whole or part of the renal outline. The renal outline is normally seen because of the difference in density of the solid organ and the surrounding fat. When blood escapes into the perirenal tissues this distinction is lost.

    (b) Loss of the psoas shadow for the same reason as the loss of renal outline.

    (c) A scoliosis of the lumbar spine concave towards the side of the lesion.

    (d) Fractures of lower ribs and lumbar transverse processes.

When the injury is subcapsular a haematoma will form in the kidney and this may have the following features: (i) a bulge in the renal outline; (ii) displacement of the upper pole of the kidney away from the lumbar spine if the haematoma is in the upper pole.

2. Intravenous pyelogram: *no ureteric compression* should be applied. The pyelograms are usually of poor quality because the patient is shocked, with a low blood pressure, and gas in the bowel obscures the pyelograms.

    (a) No pyelogram if renal damage is gross.

    (b) The pelvi-calyceal structures are disorganized as the result of a haematoma or the tear in the kidney.

    (c) Contrast may escape into the renal substance or into the perirenal tissues — conclusive evidence.

3. Ultrasound and CT will clearly show the presence of renal rupture and a perirenal haematoma. Ultrasound will not, however, demonstrate function.

4. Angiography is necessary if bleeding continues or there is no function of the kidney in order to determine whether the reno-vascular pedicle is intact.

TUBERCULOSIS

The bacilli reach the kidney via the blood stream and are deposited in the renal cortex. Tubercles are formed which enlarge and come to involve the medulla. Ulceration of these lesions into the calyces may then occur. The condition is usually bilateral.

Radiological appearances

In the early stages a pyelogram may show no abnormality but in established cases three types of change are responsible for the appearances:

1. Ulceration of pyramids causes irregularity and dilatation of calyces seen on a pyelogram (Figure 9.13a).

2. Fibrosis with strangulation of calyceal stems may produce smooth dilatation of some calyces.

3. Craggy irregular areas of calcification may be present in the kidney on a plain film. These changes may or may not all be present in a given case (Figure 9.13b).

The disease, which is often bilateral, tends to spread down along the ureter which shows areas of irregular dilatation and narrowing and sometimes of calcification. Calcification of the vas and seminal vesicles may also be seen.

Involvement of the bladder shows as a contracted bladder with possibly some irregular filling defects in the region of the ureteral orifice, somewhat resembling a tumour. There is often free vesico-ureteric reflux through the rigid open ureteric orifice.

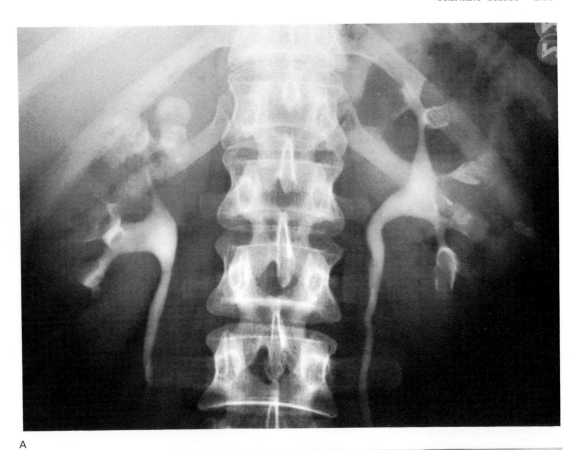

A

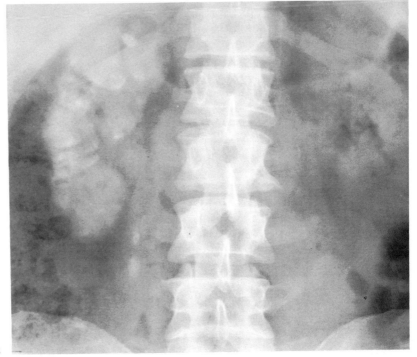

B

Fig. 9.13 Tuberculosis of kidney.
(A) IVP showing destruction and
stenosis in upper right calyces.
(B) plain radiograph showing
calcified kidney — the
tuberculous autonephrectomy.

CHRONIC PYELONEPHRITIS

This condition commonly results from vesico-ureteric reflux in infancy or childhood. Areas of inflammatory change occur in the renal substance with formation of fibrous tissue. Contraction of this fibrous tissue leads to dilatation of the nearby calyx and pulling in of the margin of the kidney.

Radiological appearances
   1. A small kidney with an irregular outline (Figure 9.14).
   2. Dilated calyces scattered throughout the kidney.
   3. Good contrast density is usually shown in a pyelogram because the contrast is excreted by hypertrophied renal tissue between the areas of scarring.
   4. If unilateral, the good kidney is large due to hypertrophy (Figure 9.15).

RENAL OPACITIES

   1. *Opaque calculi* may be single or multiple, small or large and are in the collecting system.
   2. *Calcification*: tuberculous — common — craggy, scattered in the renal substance and may be bilateral; tumour — occasionally — may be curvilinear or amorphous; cyst — rare — usually curvilinear; nephrocalcinosis — bilateral and scattered in an arc in the medulla.
   3. *Medullary sponge kidney* may be bilateral or unilateral with small opacities scattered in an arc in the medulla.
   4. *Papillary necrosis*: there may occasionally be opacities due to opaque calculi with radiolucent centres resulting from calcified freed papillae.

Urinary calculi
There are multiple causes of urinary calculi and the reader is referred to surgical texts for this information. They may be single or multiple and may be present anywhere in the urinary tract.

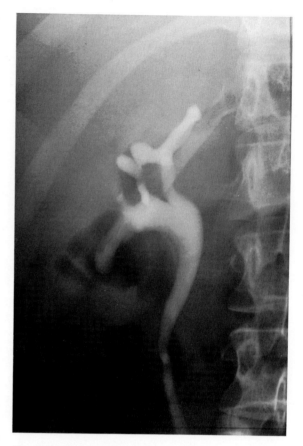

Fig. 9.14 Chronic pyelonephritis on IVP.

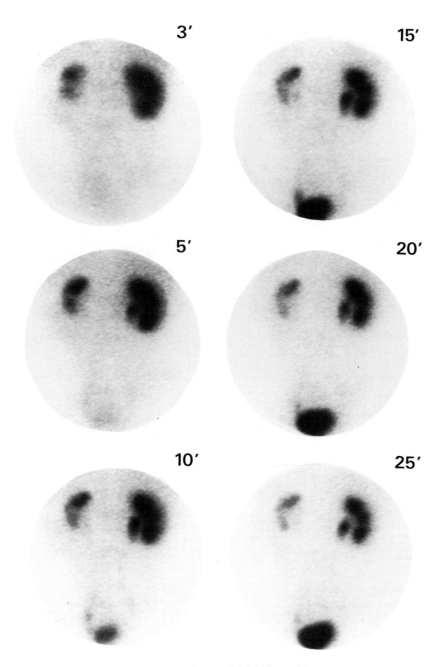

Fig. 9.15 Radionuclide renal scan showing small left kidney with reduced function in chronic pyelonephritis.

Radiologically there are three groups of calculi: (a) dense calculi; (b) calculi of intermediate density; (c) radiolucent calculi.

Dense calculi may be formed by calcium oxalate, calcium phosphate, calcium carbonate, urates, or ammonium magnesium phosphate (Figure 9.16). They appear as dense white opacities on plain films. Oxalate stones may be laminated and the large stag-horn calculi which fill the pelvi-calyceal system are usually phosphatic.

Calculi of intermediate density are composed of cystine and appear as low density opacities on plain films.

Radiolucent calculi are composed of uric acid or xanthine. They are not visible on a plain film but appear as filling defects in contrast medium.

Ureteric calculi
These are usually small and oval but may be irregular in shape.

Radiological appearances
1. Plain radiographs: if they are opaque they may be visible in the line of the ureter on plain films.
2. Intravenous pyelography: in acute obstruction of the ureter by a stone an intravenous pyelogram will show the following in the kidney on the same side as the stone: (a) delayed excretion of the contrast medium (Figure 9.17); (b) increased density of the contrast medium in the kidney; (c) prolonged opacification of the renal substance (nephrogram); (d) dilatation of the pelvis, calyces and ureter down to the site of the stone.

Because of the obstruction it may be several hours or even days before the contrast medium will extend down to the site of the block and films made over this period may be necessary to show the site of the calculus.

In more long-standing obstruction, hydronephrosis develops with marked reduction of renal function to the extent that the pelvis and calyces may not be visible on intravenous pyelograms.

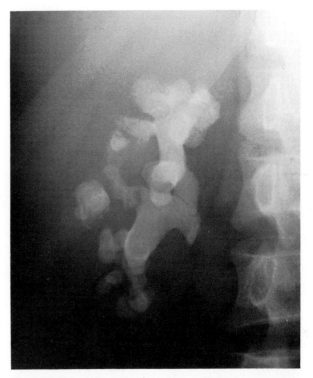

Fig. 9.16 Plain radiograph of stag-horn calculus.

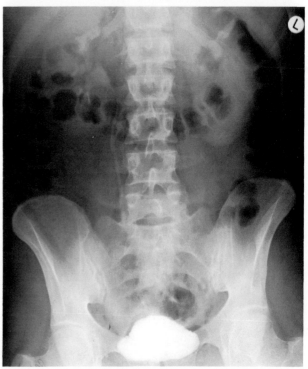

Fig. 9.17 IVP with delayed nephrogram on left due to obstruction by a left ureteric calculus.

Other valuable techniques for showing the site and effects of calculi are as follows:

3. Computerized tomography.

4. Ultrasound: in both CT and ultrasound the hydronephrosis can be seen without contrast medium and the ureteric dilatation followed in many cases down to the obstructing lesion.

5. Retrograde pyelography will locate the obstruction and by passing it, if possible, with the catheter the pressure can be relieved.

6. Nuclear medicine, because of its high sensitivity, will show not only if there is residual function, but also the degree of hydronephrosis and the level of the obstruction.

Nephrocalcinosis

There is a deposition of small collections of calcium within the renal substance (Figure 9.18). The condition is bilateral and results from two groups of causes:

1. *Hypercalcaemia and hypercalcuria*: hyperparathyroidism, multiple myeloma, secondary deposits in bone, milk-alkali syndrome, hypervitaminosis D, sarcoid, steroid therapy, renal tubular acidosis, Cushing's syndrome, idiopathic hypercalcuria, or prolonged bed rest may each be responsible for hypercalcaemia and hypercalcuria.

2. *Changes within the kidney*: medullary sponge kidney.

The kidneys are often reduced in size in group one, but normal or increased in size in medullary sponge kidney.

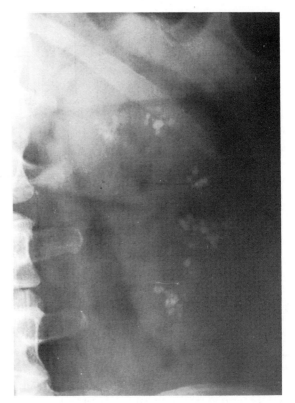

Fig. 9.18 Nephrocalcinosis on plain radiograph.

RENAL CYSTIC DISEASE

Solitary cyst

Single cysts vary in size from very small to very large and produce no symptoms. They are very common and are seen in up to 30% of abdominal CT scans without symptoms referrable to the kidneys.

Radiological appearances

1. Plain radiographs: (a) if large enough and near the surface the cyst will produce a bulge in the renal outline; (b) if centrally placed in the

kidney there may only be a generalized enlargement of the kidney; (c) calcification in the wall occurs in a small percentage of cases and is curvilinear.

2. Intravenous pyelogram (Figure 9.19): (a) displacement and stretching of calyces; (b) clubbing of calyces may occur due to pressure on the calyceal stem; (c) a round area of translucency in the nephrogram.

3. Ultrasound has largely replaced angiography in the diagnosis of cysts and the differentiation of cysts from tumours (Figure 9.20).

4. Computerized tomography: shows the presence and fluid-filled nature of the cysts, but like the other tests cannot completely exclude a small tumour *en plaque* in the cyst (Figure 9.21).

5. Angiography: (a) displacement of vessels around the cyst; (b) absence of vessels in the cyst area; (c) an area of radiolucency in the nephrogram.

6. Cyst puncture: fluid withdrawn from the cyst should be subjected to examination for malignancy by cytology. Replacement of the withdrawn fluid by contrast medium will outline the cyst and, if malignant change is present, may show irregularity of the cyst wall or a filling defect.

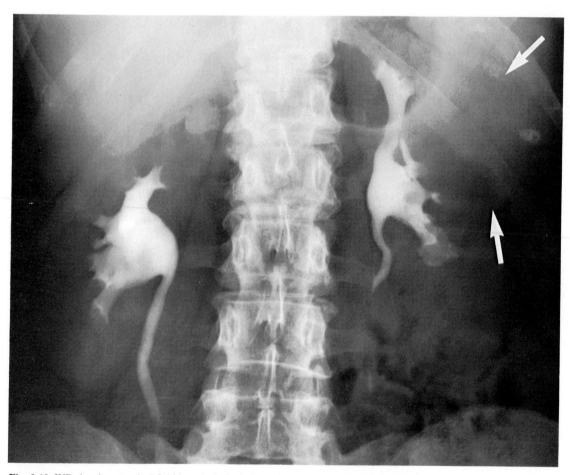

Fig. 9.19 IVP showing cyst in left kidney (→) displacing calyces.

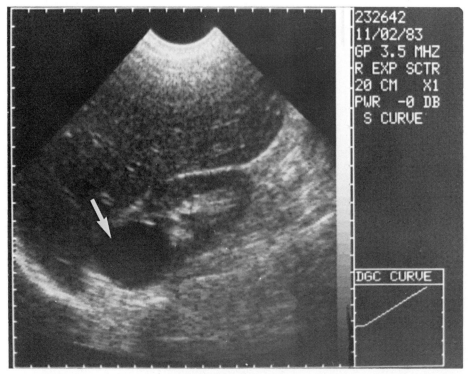

Fig. 9.20 Right renal ultrasound showing upper pole cyst (→).

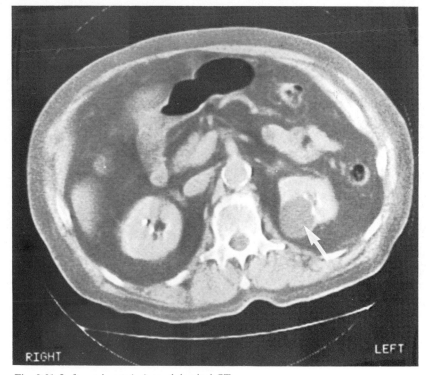

Fig. 9.21 Left renal cyst (→) on abdominal CT.

Polycystic kidneys

This congenital and familial condition is nearly
always bilateral but may affect only one kidney.
There may be cystic changes in other organs
such as the liver and pancreas.

Radiological appearances

1. Plain films: enlargement and lobulation of
the renal shadows due to projecting cysts.

2. Intravenous pyelography: (a) enlarged
lobulated kidneys; (b) stretching of the calyces
and calyceal stems; (c) calyces stretched around
cysts are large, crescentic and sharply defined.

3. Retrograde pyelography may be necessary
if the renal function is so diminished that
insufficient contrast is excreted to outline the
pelvis and calyces in an intravenous pyelogram.
The changes seen are as described under
intravenous pyelography (Figure 9.22).

4. Ultrasound and CT demonstrate well the
number, size, shape and nature of the cysts and
no further radiological examinations are usually
necessary (Figure 9.23).

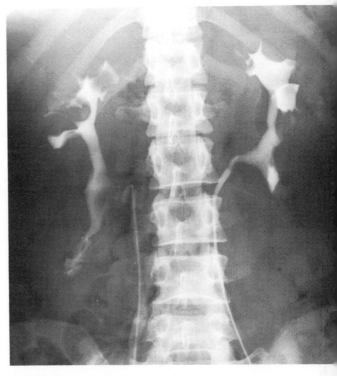

Fig. 9.22 Bilateral polycystic disease of kidneys shown by
retrograde pyelography.

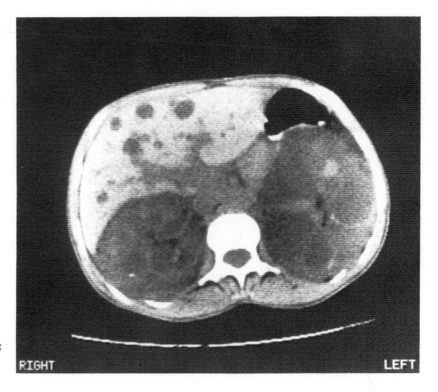

Fig. 9.23 Abdominal CT showing
polycystic disease of kidneys and
liver.

BENIGN RENAL TUMOURS

There are a number of benign tumours, such as adenoma and lipoma, but they are all rare. The haemangioma is also rare but is important since it may cause haematuria.

MALIGNANT TUMOURS

Adenocarcinoma (Grawitz) is the most common and often metastasises to lung or, less commonly, to bone, liver and brain. Nephroblastoma (Wilms) is rare but important in children.

Adenocarcinoma

Radiological appearances

1. Plain radiographs: (a) a bulge on the renal outline if the tumour is large enough and peripherally placed; (b) generalized enlargement of the kidney in large centrally placed tumours; (c) irregular and rarely linear calcification occurs occasionally.

2. Intravenous pyelogram: (a) small tumours may produce little change but larger tumours displace, stretch and *destroy* calyceal stems and calyces; (b) obstruction of calyceal stems by pressure may cause dilatation of some calyces.

3. Ultrasound: a mass is seen displacing calyces and distorting the parenchyma. It will distinguish cystic from solid masses.

4. Computerized tomography: renal masses are clearly shown together with the density of the contents, differentiating solid from cystic masses (Figure 9.24).

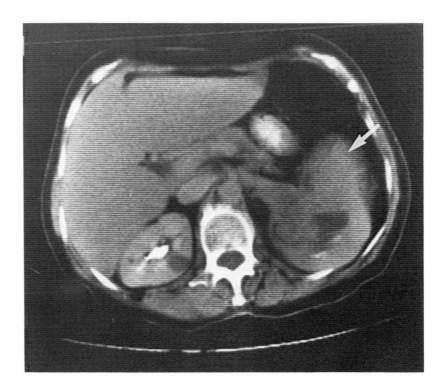

Fig. 9.24 Left renal carcinoma shown by abdominal CT (→).

5. Angiography. This usually distinguishes between cyst and tumour since cysts are avascular and tumours in the majority of cases show abnormal tumour vessels within the mass (Figure 9.25).

'Skinny needle' (22 gauge) biopsy under CT or ultrasound control is now an accepted method of cytological diagnosis.

Nephroblastoma (Wilms' tumour)

This tumour occurs almost exclusively in young children, 70% of cases occurring under the age of 3 years and 90% under the age of 5 years.

Radiological appearances

1. Plain radiographs: (a) a soft tissue mass is present in the renal area; (b) calcification may occasionally be present in the mass.

2. Intravenous pyelography: (a) destruction of some calyces (Figure 9.26); (b) displacement and stretching of some calyces; (c) the renal pelvis may be stretched over the tumour mass.

3. Ultrasound: the tumour is shown in the renal area and local invasion may be demonstrated.

4. Computerized tomography: this also shows the tumour and local spread or node involvement.

Metastases from the tumour are most frequently found in the lungs. Occasionally there are osteolytic metastases in bone. Nephroblastoma must be distinguished from neuroblastoma arising in the adrenal, which also occurs in young children. On plain films a distinction between them may not be possible, although the neuroblastoma is more commonly calcified than the nephroblastoma.

On intravenous pyelography the whole kidney may be seen to be displaced by a neuroblastoma; this is also shown by ultrasound and CT (see 'Tumours of the adrenal' page 247), and distinguishes between a neuroblastoma and a nephroblastoma.

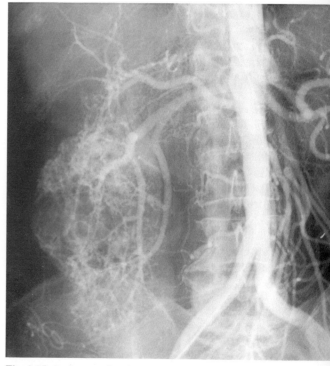

Fig. 9.25 Angiogram showing hypervascularity and distortion due to right renal carcinoma.

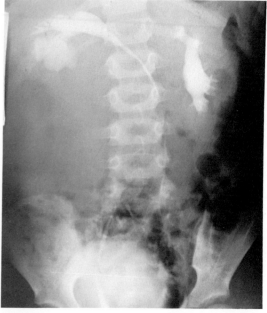

Fig. 9.26 IVP showing displacement and distortion of right pelvi-calyceal system by a Wilms' tumour of the right kidney.

PELVIC AND URETERIC TUMOURS

Benign tumours
These are rare and radiologically
indistinguishable from malignant neoplasms.

Malignant tumours
Carcinoma of the renal pelvis presents in an
intravenous or retrograde pyelogram as an
irregular filling defect or as irregularity of the
margin of the pelvis due to ulceration. The
tumour sometimes seeds along the ureter and
into the bladder, resulting in other tumours at
these sites. Carcinoma of the ureter may present
as either an irregular stricture or sometimes as a
local dilatation of the ureter to accommodate the
mass of the tumour.

Differential diagnosis
1. Blood clot in the renal pelvis.
2. A non-opaque calculus.

RENAL MASSES
A suggested sequence of imaging investigations for
a renal mass is shown in Diagnostic decision tree
8b, page 307.

PAPILLARY NECROSIS

This condition occurs in diabetes urinary
tract obstruction, and with phenacetin abuse,
and results from ischaemia of the pyramids.
Several pyramids are usually affected in both
kidneys. The appearances in the early stages
may be difficult to distinguish from tuberculosis.
The kidney is usually reduced in size but is
smooth in contour.

Radiological appearances (Figure 9.27)
   1. Small smooth kidney.
   2. Irregularly or smoothly dilated calyces.
   3. Papillae lying free in the calyces and
producing filling defects may be seen in a
pyelogram.
   4. Calculi with a characteristic radiolucent
centre may be present.

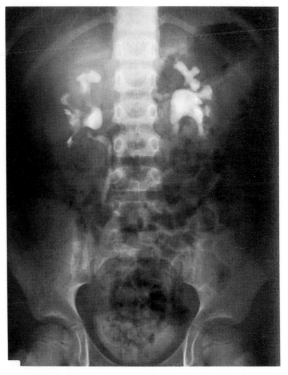

Fig. 9.27 Papillary necrosis on IVP.

RENO-VASCULAR HYPERTENSION

Renal ischaemia as a cause of hypertension may arise from:

1. Stenosis or obstruction of major or segmental renal arteries by either atheroma or fibromuscular hyperplasia.

2. Localized renal ischaemia associated with previous infection, trauma, or pressure from cysts.

3. Generalized renal parenchymal disease such as pyelonephritis.

Establishment of a renal cause and differentiation of the pathological causes is important in the treatment. Vessel narrowing may be surgically or interventionally remediable or unilateral renal parenchymal disease may indicate nephrectomy.

Pyelonephritis and cystic disease are detailed on pages 262 and 268 respectively.

Radiological investigations

1. Intravenous pyelography. The significant findings are as follows:

(a) Small kidney. A difference in renal lengths of more than 2 cm is regarded as significant.

(b) Reduced cortical thickness. Minimum normal is 1 cm (see 'interpapillary line', page 253).

(c) Scarring producing irregularity of the renal outline. Indicative of previous disease, possibly infarcts.

(d) Slow excretion relative to the normal side.

(e) High concentration relative to the normal side.

(f) Slow washout with induced diuresis (usually intravenous Lasix).

2. Renal angiography, although usually performed by aortic catheterization, may now be done by the digital subtraction technique with an intravenous injection. Stenosis of the renal arteries may be shown due to atheroma or fibromuscular hyperplasia (Figure 9.28). Segmental hypoperfusion may also be shown and may result from previous vascular or parenchymal lesions.

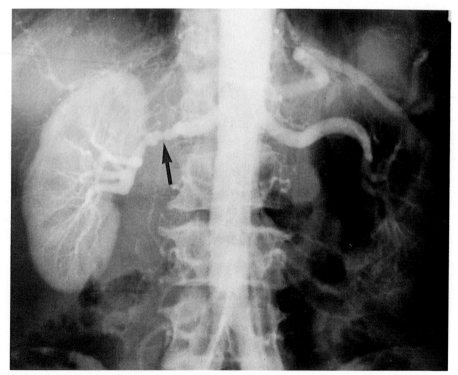

Fig. 9.28 Renal angiogram demonstrating stenosis of right renal artery by fibromuscular hyperplasia.

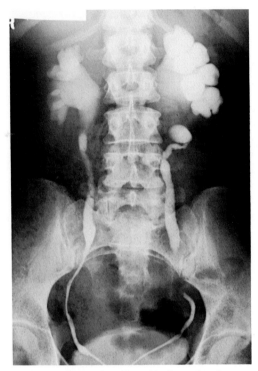

Fig. 9.29 IVP showing bilateral hydronephrosis due to retroperitoneal fibrosis.

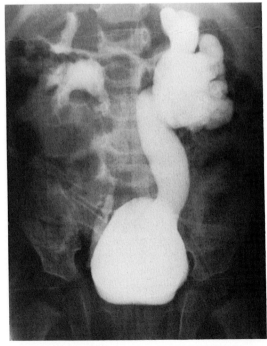

Fig. 9.30 Gross left vesico-ureteric reflux, and mild right reflux, at cysto-urethrogram.

3. Renal venous sampling is performed by selective catheterization of renal veins via the femoral vein and inferior vena cava. The samples are analysed for renin levels to localize, if possible, the site of renin production.

4. Radionuclide scanning may show differential renal perfusion between the two kidneys but is not as useful as venous sampling and angiography.

THE URETERS

PERI-URETERIC FIBROSIS
Although a disease of unknown origin, it has followed the use of methysergide for the treatment of migraine and is characterized by the formation of fibrous tissue in the retroperitoneal area. The fibrosis causes narrowing and medial displacement of usually both ureters with obstruction to urine flow (Figure 9.29).

VESICO-URETERIC REFLUX
Reflux is normally prevented by a valvular mechanism at the vesico-ureteric junction, due to the oblique course of the ureter through the bladder wall. When this mechanism breaks down bladder contents may enter the ureters.

There are many causes, such as congenital abnormalities of the vesico-ureteric junction, ectopic ureter, ureterocele, double ureter, cystitis, lower tract obstruction, tuberculosis, and carcinoma of the bladder, but the most common reflux is idiopathic. Idiopathic reflux may occur in young children and disappear as they grow older, and is frequently responsible for the development of reflux nephropathy.

Radiological appearances
Micturating cysto-urethrogram: reflux may be seen by fluoroscopy when the bladder is filled with contrast medium and the patient strains or micturates. The contrast may enter only the lower part of the ureter, or may fill the ureter, pelvis and calyces (Figure 9.30). The ureters and pelvi-calyceal structures are usually dilated, but may be normal in appearance.

THE BLADDER

BLADDER TUMOURS

These may arise in the bladder or be the result of seeding from a tumour higher up in the urinary tract. It is not possible to distinguish between innocent and malignant tumours radiologically. Double contrast cystography using a combination of contrast medium and gas in the bladder may show small tumours better than ordinary cystography.

Radiological appearances

1. Cystography: (a) there may be a lobulated or irregular filling defect (Figure 9.31); (b) there may only be an area of irregularity of the bladder wall.

2. Computerized tomography is the radiological examination of choice for staging bladder tumours, since it will show not only the size and shape of the mass but also any extension through the wall, and lymphatic metastases in the pelvic and para-aortic nodes (Figure 9.32).

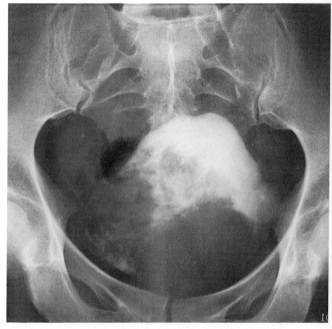

Fig. 9.31 Cystogram showing large irregular filling defect of bladder carcinoma.

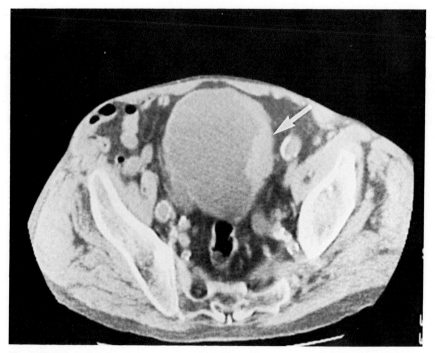

Fig. 9.32 Pelvic CT showing thickening of bladder wall by carcinoma (→).

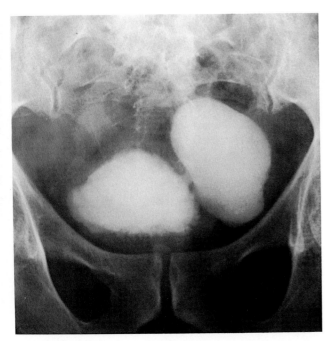

Fig. 9.33 Cystogram showing bladder and large left-sided diverticulum.

DIVERTICULA

These are usually the result of lower urinary tract obstruction, and may be single or multiple, small or very large (Figure 9.33). They are best demonstrated by voiding cysto-urethrography, when they become more apparent than on an ordinary cystogram.

NEUROGENIC BLADDER

There are many causes of a neurogenic bladder, such as spinal cord trauma, disseminated sclerosis, diabetes and tabes. It may also occur after pelvic operations.

Radiological appearances
Appearances vary and there may be one of the following:

1. Marked atony of a large, thin-walled bladder which does not undergo contraction.

2. A small, thick-walled bladder which has the shape of a 'fir tree'.

These appearances are often associated with dilatation of the upper urinary tract.

THE PROSTATE

ENLARGED PROSTATE

It is not possible to tell from the radiological appearances whether prostatic enlargement is benign hypertophy or the result of carcinoma. The presence of sclerotic metastases in the skeletal pelvis will, of course, suggest carcinoma.

Radiological appearances
Early:

1. A smooth, convex or sometimes lobulated filling defect in the base of the bladder in the cystogram (Figure 9.34).

2. Elongation of the prostatic urethra shown by urethrography.

Later:

3. A trabeculated bladder wall, often with diverticula.

4. Dilatation of the upper urinary tract.

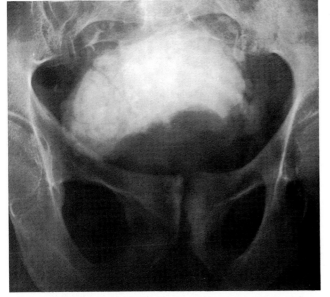

Fig. 9.34 Prostatic impression on floor of bladder, shown at I.V.P.

5. The lower ends of the ureters are often the shape of a fish hook due to elevation of the bladder floor.

6. Residual urine in the bladder after micturition.

Enlarged prostate may be well shown on magnetic resonance imaging (Figure 9.35).

Carcinoma of the prostate is particularly prone to metastasise to bone. Such metastases are seen on: (a) radiographs — sclerotic deposits; (b) radionuclide bone scan — very high activity lesions.

Assessment of the progress of hormonal treatment of prostatic metastases is usually by biochemistry and nuclear medicine bone scanning.

PROSTATIC CALCULI
Collections of small dense opacities within the prostate may be seen on a plain film and represent calculi.

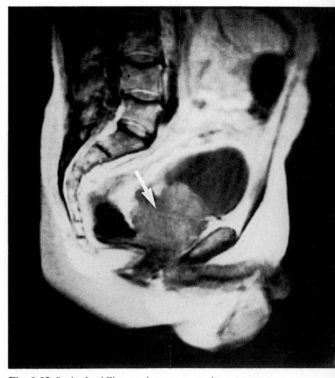

Fig. 9.35 Sagittal midline section on magnetic resonance imaging showing large prostate projecting into floor of bladder (Philips Gyroscan, by courtesy of Philips Medical Systems Div, Eindhoven, The Netherlands).

THE URETHRA

URETHRAL OBSTRUCTION
There are a variety of causes of urethral obstruction included amongst which are prostatic enlargement, urethral valves, Marion's disease, urethral stricture, meatal stenosis, neurogenic causes and calculus.

Radiological appearances
The results of urethral obstruction vary with the degree and length of time of the obstruction.
Early:
1. Dilatation of the urethra above the obstruction and seen on voiding cysto-urethrography.
2. Trabeculation and diverticula in the bladder shown on a cystogram.
Later:
3. Ureteric and pelvi-calyceal dilatation.
4. Vesico-ureteric reflux.
5. Narrowing of the renal cortex.
6. Changes of reflux nephropathy.

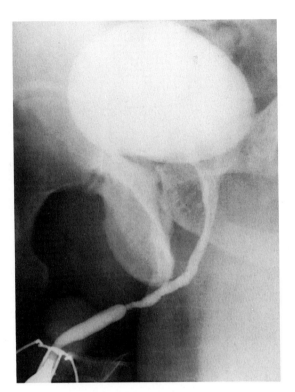

Fig. 9.36 Inflammatory urethral stricture shown by retrograde urethrography.

Urethral valves
See congenital abnormalities (page 258).

Urethral stricture
Congenital urethral strictures form a small group but the majority of strictures result from infection or trauma (Figure 9.36). Neoplasm is an occasional cause. They may be multiple, show as narrowing of the lumen and are best shown by micturating cysto-urethrography.

HAEMATURIA
Haematuria is a common and important presenting sign of pathology in any part of the urinary tract. A suggested sequence of imaging investigations for this sign is shown in Diagnostic decision tree 8a, page 307.

10 Reproductive System

Obstetrics

METHODS OF INVESTIGATION

Radiography
Due to the potential damaging effects of radiation on the growing fetus, radiography is used during pregnancy only on strong indications.

Ultrasound
In obstetrics this is the imaging procedure of choice. The safety of ultrasound is a major factor.

Computerized tomography
This examination is of value in pelvimetry but is otherwise rarely used.

Magnetic resonance imaging
In the future this may well become useful as a radiationless procedure.

Hysterosalpingography
The uterine cavity and fallopian tubes are outlined by contrast medium injected via the cervix.

NORMAL PREGNANCY

There is considerable debate as to whether all pregnancies should be checked by ultrasound to establish normality or otherwise. If the examination is performed it is desirable to carry it out before 20 weeks gestation, the latest time for performing a relatively simple abortion (Figure 10.1). Ultrasound will rapidly establish the following points:

1. The presence of a gestation and whether it is intra-uterine or extra-uterine.

2. The period of gestation, the accuracy varying from $\pm$ 4 days in early pregnancy, to $\pm$ 4 weeks near term.

3. Whether it is a single or multiple pregnancy (Figure 10.2).

4. The presence of a fetal heartbeat which indicates fetal viability. Heartbeat is usually visible after 5 weeks' gestation.

5. The presence of normal organogenesis of the skeleton, brain, liver, kidneys, bladder and spine.

6. The situation and state of the placenta.

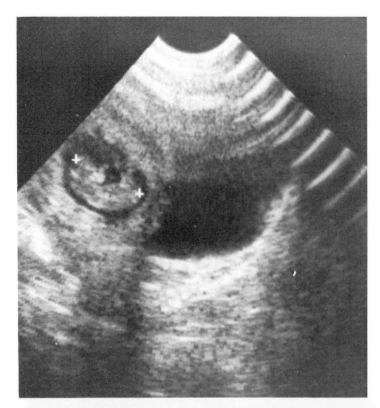

Fig. 10.1 Normal ultrasound of eight week gestation.

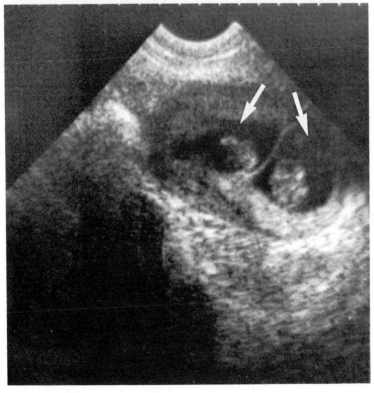

Fig. 10.2 Twin pregnancy showing two amniotic sacs, at eight weeks gestation (→).

ABNORMAL PREGNANCY

FETAL ABNORMALITIES

Only major anomalies in development can be detected antenatally by ultrasound, although the use of amniocentesis and measurement of alpha-fetoprotein provides a sensitive test for neural tube defects.

The following groups of abnormalities may be demonstrated by ultrasound:

Cranial and spinal defects (Figure 10.3)
These include hydrocephalus, and all the degrees of rachischisis. In late pregnancy confirmation by radiography is useful.

Genito-urinary defects
Conditions such as Potter's syndrome with absence of kidneys and bladder, or urethral valves with bladder, ureteric and calyceal dilatation, are all well shown especially in late pregnancy (Figure 10.4). Failure of passage of urine into the amniotic sac usually produces oligohydramnios.

Gastrointestinal abnormalities
Amongst these are oesophageal, duodenal or intestinal atresias. Dilatation of the gut proximal to an obstruction may be seen ('double bubble' in duodenal atresia). Failure to swallow and absorb amniotic fluid may give rise to polyhydramnios.

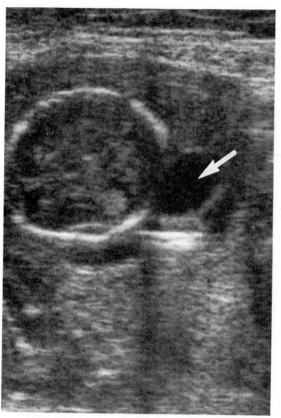

Fig. 10.3 Ultrasound of fetal head at 16 weeks gestation, showing fluid-filled encephalocele (→).

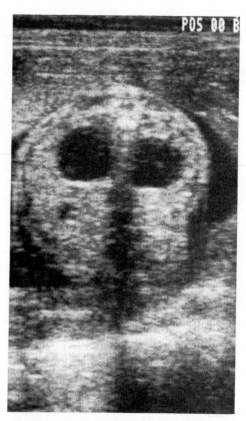

Fig. 10.4 Ultrasound cross-section of fetal abdomen at 28 weeks gestation, showing hydronephrotic kidneys (→).

Diaphragmatic hernia
Gut may be shown in the fetal thorax.

Abnormalities of limbs
Abnormalities may be seen if looked for carefully.

Conjoined twins ('Siamese twins')
This condition is rare but diagnosable.

Fetal death
There is lack of heartbeat and limb movement. Fetal oedema (Figure 10.5) and sometimes Spalding's sign (overlapping skull bones) may be seen by both ultrasound and radiography.

Immune disorders
Rh incompatibility may show fetal oedema, pleural or peritoneal effusions, and polyhydramnios.

Fetal developmental retardation
This is probably due to placental insufficiency, and shows either as delayed growth of the head and body, or as principally affecting the body. If established, it is an indication for early delivery.

Blighted ovum
Early failure of fetal development shows ultrasonographically as a small-for-dates amniotic sac, without a live fetal pole or with no fetal pole.

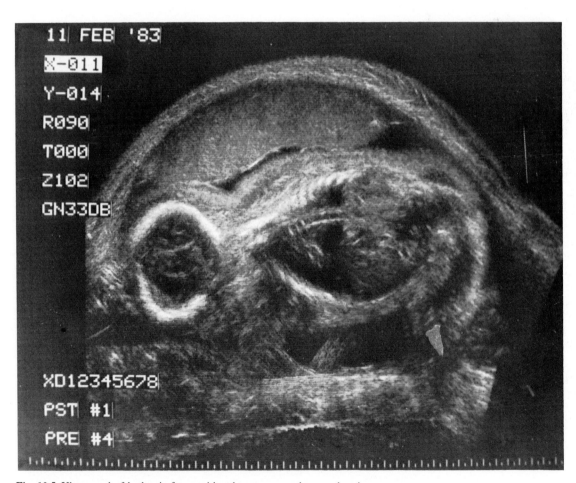

Fig. 10.5 Ultrasound of hydropic fetus, with subcutaneous oedema and ascites.

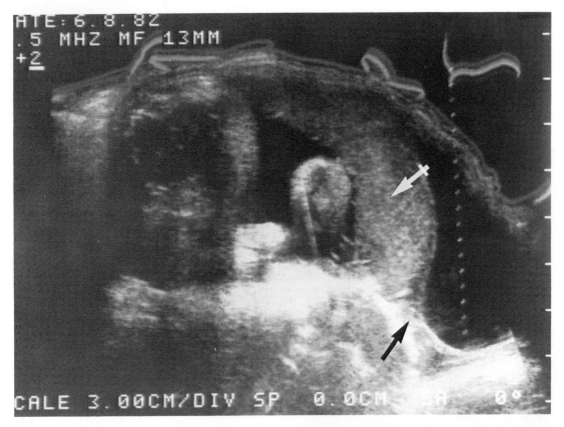

Fig. 10.6 Ultrasound of placenta praevia, showing position of internal cervical os (→) and placenta (↔).

PLACENTAL ABNORMALITIES

Antepartum haemorrhage is usually due to retroplacental bleeding. Ultrasound will establish whether the fetus is still viable, whether the placenta is praevia, or whether a haematoma or other abnormality is present. The most important anomaly is placenta praevia (Figure 10.6), and this is usually easily diagnosed by ultrasound, which shows the size, consistency and position of the placenta reliably. Placental degeneration, hydatidiform mole or choriocarcinoma are also well seen on ultrasound (Figure 10.7).

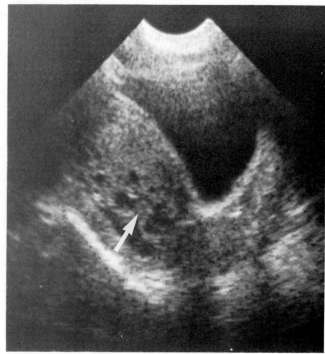

Fig. 10.7 Ultrasound of hydatidiform mole. Cysts in mole (→).

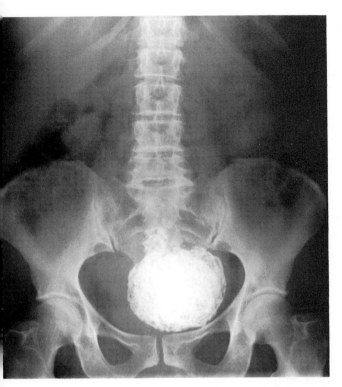

Fig. 10.8 Calcified fibroid in abdominal radiograph.

UTERINE ABNORMALITIES
The presence of congenital abnormalities of the maternal uterus are not evident during pregnancy unless they are a gross condition such as a septate uterus. Fibroids may complicate a pregnancy by either degeneration or obstruction of delivery, and are well seen on ultrasound or, if calcified, on radiographs (Figure 10.8).

EXTRA-UTERINE PREGNANCY
Ectopic pregnancy usually presents with pain and perhaps bleeding. Ultrasound will establish if the gestation is intra-uterine, or if it is not, will often show the extra-uterine site together with any free fluid in the pouch of Douglas (Figure 10.9). Later in pregnancy a viable extra-uterine fetus may be seen in the peritoneal cavity separate from the uterus.

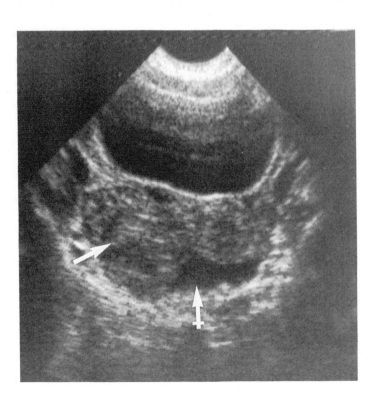

Fig. 10.9 Transverse ultrasound of ruptured ectopic pregnancy. Ectopic gestation (→); fluid in pouch of Douglas (↔).

SPONTANEOUS ABORTION

Ultrasound readily demonstrates whether a viable fetus is still *in utero* and the amniotic sac is still present or, if there has been loss of products of conception, whether there is any debris still in the uterine cavity (Figure 10.10).

PELVIMETRY

This is used to measure the size of the maternal pelvis prior to or during pregnancy, to estimate the probability of vaginal delivery. Multiple radiographic views are required for proper assessment of the bony pelvis. Computerized tomography has a definite place in producing equivalent information with less radiation.

FERTILITY STUDIES

Ultrasound may assist in fertility studies by showing the development of Graafian follicles in the ovaries, and thus allowing an estimate of the optimal times for intercourse to produce conception or for the collection of ova for *in vitro* fertilization.

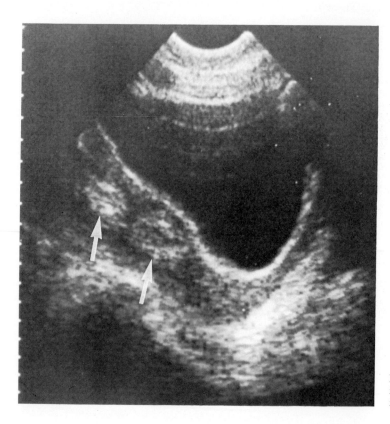

Fig. 10.10 Ultrasound of incomplete abortion, with debris in uterine cavity (→).

Gynaecology

UTERUS

CONGENITAL LESIONS

Hypoplasia or degrees of septation of the uterus
are uncommon and usually present with
difficulties in pregnancy. Ultrasound may show
major degrees of these conditions but
hysterography shows them best (Figure 10.11).

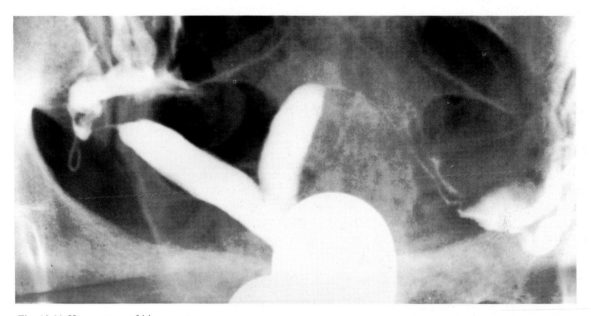

Fig. 10.11 Hysterogram of bicornuate uterus.

BENIGN MASSES

Fibroids are relatively common and are best seen
on ultrasound, where they appear as echogenic
single or multiple masses in or protruding from
the myometrium. Degeneration during
pregnancy may cause pain. Calcification in
fibroids is frequently seen on plain films of the
pelvis (see Figure 10.8)

MALIGNANT MASSES

Tumours generally arise in either the
endometrium or cervix. Ultrasound may show
enlargement of the uterus, but the most useful
imaging examination is CT, which shows not
only the size and shape of the uterus, but
extension of the tumour into the pelvic soft
tissues and lateral pelvic lymph nodes.

FALLOPIAN TUBES

The most common lesion of the fallopian tubes is occlusion, resulting in infertility either accidentally or by intent (surgically). Hydrosalpinx or pyosalpinx may be seen on ultrasound as a fluid-filled, or semi-solid mass adjacent to the uterus, and is often difficult to differentiate from ovarian masses. Hystero-salpingography will show obstruction or patency of the tubes (Figure 10.12) and, if communicating, a hydrosalpinx.

OVARIES

The ovaries are normally seen by ultrasound, together with the normal cycle of follicular development.

CONGENITAL ANOMALIES
Abnormalities in size are rare but may be seen by ultrasound.

CYSTS
Ovarian cysts may be normal follicular or corpus luteum cysts, but large solitary cysts or multiple cysts do occur. These are well seen on both ultrasound and CT (Figure 10.13).

TUMOURS
Ovarian tumours may be cystic, as in the case of the cystadenoma, or solid, as in teratomas, sarcomas and carcinomas. Ultrasound and CT show the size, shape and consistency of the masses well. Plain radiographs will also show cysts if calcification is present (Figure 10.14).

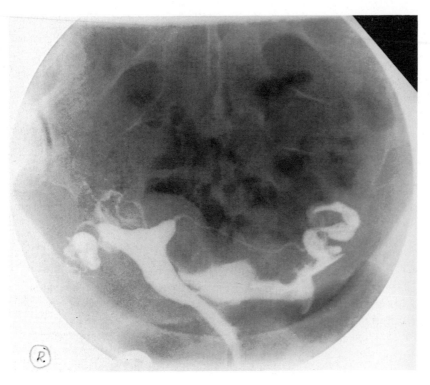

Fig. 10.12 Normal hysterogram showing patent Fallopian tubes.

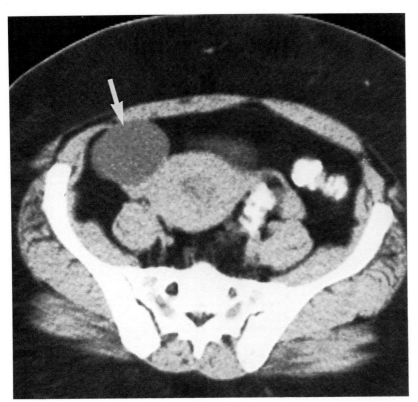

Fig. 10.13 CT showing cyst ($\rightarrow$) in ovary.

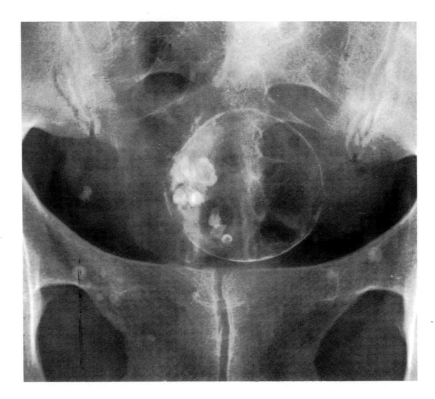

Fig. 10.14 Dermoid cyst of ovary containing rudimentary teeth.

The breast

METHODS OF INVESTIGATION

Radiography
There are two major methods:
1. *Film mammography*, utilizing single emulsion high resolution film and very low kV x-rays.
2. *Xeromammography*, which is a dry process based on the semiconductor properties of selenium; this very high contrast technique is a popular method of showing soft tissues of breast and other areas (see Chapter 1).
Normal appearances (Figure 10.15):
1. The skin thickness is uniform and there is no tethering of the skin to underlying structures.
2. The breast tissue varies markedly in quantity and density between individuals, over the menstrual cycle, and from menarche, through reproductive life to the post-menopausal stage. The probability of neoplasm appears to rise with increasing density.
3. The underlying muscle planes and ribs are visible.
4 Lymph nodes may be visible in the axilla.

Ductography
Contrast medium is injected into the lactiferous ducts and films made showing the opacified ducts.

Ultrasound
This has in general been used only to demonstrate whether a palpable or radiographic mass is solid or cystic, but with the development of specialized equipment it is becoming a significant tool for diagnosis.

Thermography
Unfortunately the nature of the lesion causing superficial temperature variation cannot be specifically determined and the technique is now little used.

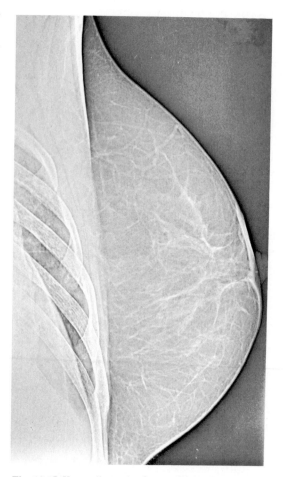

Fig. 10.15 Xeroradiograph of normal breast.

THE ROLES OF BREAST IMAGING

1. To act as a survey mechanism in women (rarely in men) to detect or exclude the presence of carcinoma.
2. To help differentiate between benign and malignant disease in clinically abnormal breasts.
3. In proven breast neoplasm, to assist with staging, to improve management and to provide objective follow-up and assessment of treatment.

Currently the major imaging test is mammography using either film or xeroradiography.

LESIONS OF THE BREAST

TRAUMA
Direct injury occasionally results in fat necrosis with the appearance of coarse calcifications on mammography.

CYSTIC HYPERPLASIA
This relatively common condition must be differentiated from carcinoma.

Radiological appearances
   1. Mammography shows relatively dense irregular stroma, usually with multiple areas of uniform density with smooth margins due to cysts, which may be fluid-filled or contain solid

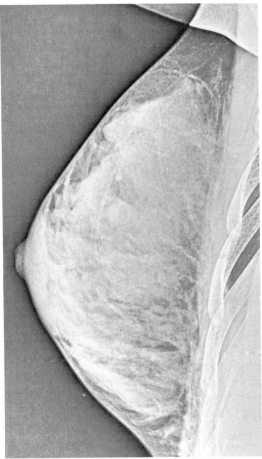

Fig. 10.16 Xeroradiograph of breast with extensive mammary dysplasia.

material (Figure 10.16). Calcification, if present, is coarse and irregular.
   2. Ultrasound: fluid-filled cysts may be shown (Figure 10.17). This does not exclude neoplasm, but lowers the probability markedly.

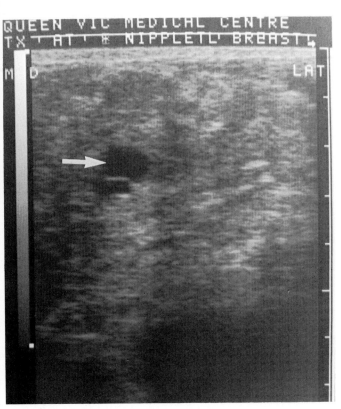

Fig. 10.17 Ultrasound of mammary dysplasia showing cyst.

FIBRO-ADENOMA

This usually occurs in young women as single or multiple masses.

Radiological appearances

1. Mammography usually shows a relatively dense stroma with a well-defined mass, no fibrous extensions and no skin involvement.

2. Ultrasound shows the mass to be solid. Carcinoma cannot be excluded by imaging methods and excision biopsy is required.

CARCINOMA

Most primary neoplasms of breast are either infiltrative or intraductal. In most cases, a palpable mass or nipple bleeding will be present. In a significant number of cases mammography will demonstrate an occult lesion in a clinically normal breast.

Radiological appearances

1. Mammography (Figure 10.18). The classic signs are as follows:
    (a) Calcification, usually of the so-called 'broken needle' type, i.e. fine, irregular and multiple. In duct carcinoma it tends to lie along the lines of the ducts affected.
    (b) A mass with irregular spiculated borders.
    (c) Coarse tissue strands extending to the skin or deep muscles from a mass with perhaps dimpling of the skin.
    (d) Thickening of the skin and subcutaneous tissues.
    (e) Enlargement of axillary lymph nodes.

2. Ultrasound: one or more irregular solid masses may be seen in the breast. If the mass is not palpable, it may be localized with a needle under radiographic control to enable accurate biopsy.

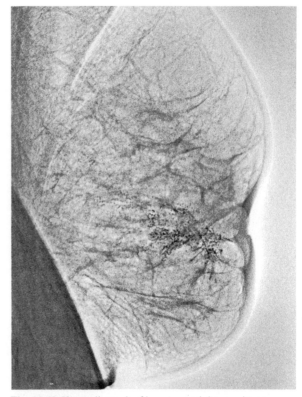

Fig. 10.18 Xeroradiograph of breast containing carcinoma. Note the calcification.

Staging of a proven breast neoplasm is important for management and involves (a) chest radiographs to check for lung metastases, (b) a radionuclide bone scan to check for metastases, and (c) A radionuclide liver scan to check for metastases.

Should signs and symptoms suggest mediastinal or cerebral involvement, CT scanning of the appropriate areas is indicated since it is the most sensitive and specific method of detection of such metastases available.

The testis

METHODS OF INVESTIGATION

Ultrasound
High resolution, small parts ultrasound produces excellent images of the scrotum and its contents. The body of the testis normally produces relatively uniform echoes, with the epididymis visible alongside (Figure 10.19).

Radionuclide scan
This is useful only to demonstrate relative vascularity of the testes, although some work has been done on locating undescended testes by using selective radiopharmaceuticals.

Computerized tomography
Although this is infrequently used to investigate the testes themselves, it is a major tool in looking for pelvic and para-aortic neoplastic extension.

Testicular venography
Catheterization of testicular veins via the inferior vena cava is used to check for reflux in cases of varicoceles.

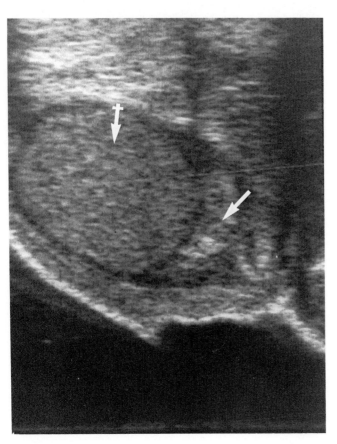

Fig. 10.19 Ultrasound of normal scrotum. Testis (↔); epididymis (→).

LESIONS OF THE TESTIS

INFECTION AND TORSION

Acute testicular pain in a boy is usually due to either infection or torsion. Radionuclide flow studies will show either reduced blood flow to the affected side, indicating torsion, or increased flow suggesting inflammation.

NEOPLASMS

An enlarged testis may be due to infection or tumour.

Radiological appearances

1. Ultrasound will show the presence or absence of hydrocele (Figure 10.20), and differentiate between an abnormality of the testis proper or of the epididymis. Tumours of the testis itself may be seen while still quite small, e.g. 3–4 mm in diameter. These are usually seminomas or teratomas.

2. Computerized tomography is valuable in the case of tumours to assess extension along the vas deferens and associated structures, as well as lymph node involvement in the pelvic and para-aortic regions.

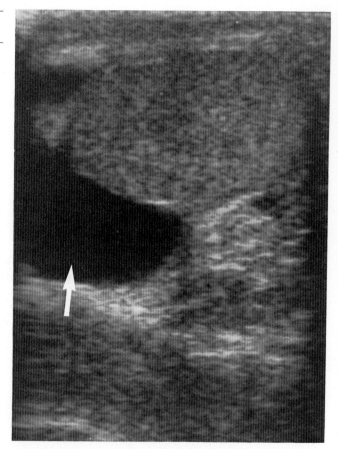

Fig. 10.20 Ultrasound of scrotum showing testis and hydrocele (→).

11 Interventional Radiology

Interventional radiology is primarily therapeutic as opposed to diagnostic and may be subdivided into several main groups:

1. Guided biopsy and/or localization of masses.

2. Abscess drainage.

3. Drainage and/or stenting of hollow viscera such as bile ducts or the urinary tract.

4. Vascular procedures including dilatation of stenosed vessels and embolization of abnormal or bleeding vessels.

GUIDED BIOPSY

The lesion, usually a tumour, once seen and located by the most appropriate imaging test — fluoroscopy, radiography, CT or ultrasound — is biopsied percutaneously using either the fine needle technique producing cytological specimens, or by cutting needles producing histological specimens. It is now common to biopsy masses in lung, bone, liver, kidney, pancreas and breast. Particularly in the breast, a guide needle or wire may be left with the tip in the mass to guide the surgeon to the correct location (Figure 11.1) in those cases where the mass can be seen on imaging but is not palpable.

ABSCESS DRAINAGE

Abscesses in most areas are usually localized by imaging tests. In cases in which percutaneous drainage is appropriate, a needle and then a drain tube can be introduced under imaging control, thus avoiding the necessity of surgical intervention (Figure 11.2)

VISCERAL DRAINAGE AND/OR STENTING

In cases of obstruction of the main bile ducts or the ureter, especially by neoplasms, operative relief of the obstruction may not be possible or desirable. Percutaneous cannulation of the dilated bile ducts or renal pelvis allows free drainage of bile and urine respectively (Figure 11.3). It may in some cases be possible to push a stent through the stenotic lesion into the duodenum or the bladder respectively, which produces internal drainage with maintenance of liver or renal functions (see Figure 5.19).

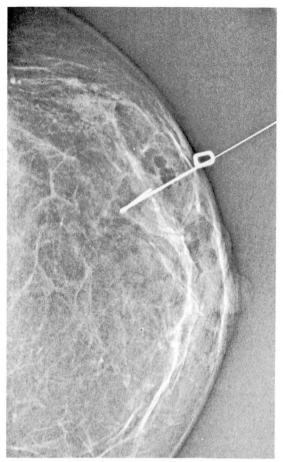

Fig. 11.1 Localisation of breast carcinoma, prior to biopsy.

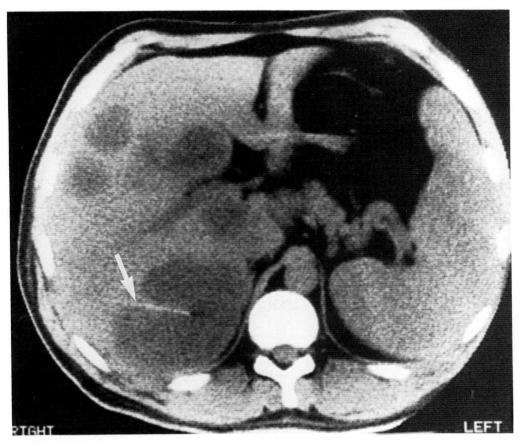

Fig. 11.2 Percutaneous drainage of liver abscess, under CT control, showing drainage catheter in abscess (→).

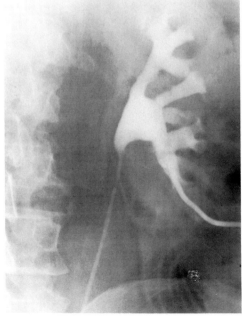

Fig. 11.3 Percutaneous nephrostomy, with antegrade pyelogram. Drainage catheter in situ.

VASCULAR PROCEDURES

Arterial stenoses in vessels to limbs, kidney and gut may be dilated by a percutaneous approach using either Dotter dilators or Gruntzig balloon catheters. The balloon catheter is an intra-arterial catheter with a balloon on its end. The deflated balloon is placed in position at the site of the stenosis under x-ray guidance and is then inflated to produce dilatation of the stenosis (Figure 11.4). This is particularly appropriate in solitary or localized stenoses, or in patients unfit for major reconstructive vascular surgery. It is usually highly effective and can be repeated if re-stenosis occurs.

Vascular tumours or arteriovenous communications may be devascularized or occluded by embolization with appropriate materials, including spring wires, balloons, super glue, or plastic particles introduced into the feeding arteries via a percutaneous catheter. The technique is used particularly in the reduction of vascularity of tumours pre-operatively, occlusion of vessels producing haemorrhage into the gut or bladder, or in arteriovenous malformations.

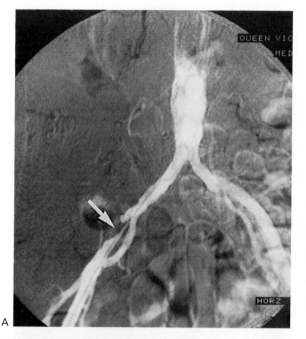

A

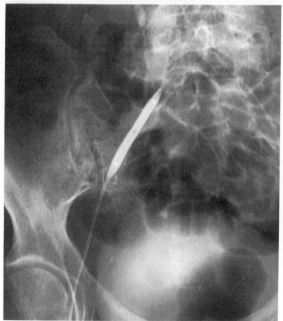

B

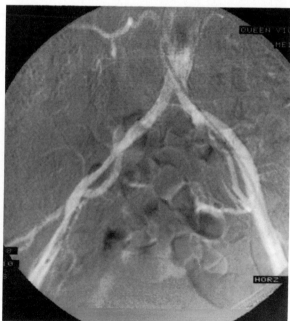

C

Fig. 11.4 Percutaneous angioplasty (balloon dilatation) of arterial stenosis.
(A) Angiogram before dilatation showing iliac stenosis (→).
(B) Balloon dilated. (C) Post dilatation angiogram.

Appendix

Diagnostic decision tree 1

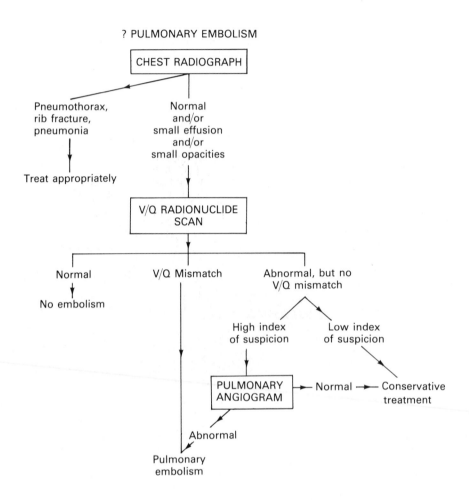

? PULMONARY EMBOLISM

CHEST RADIOGRAPH

Pneumothorax,
rib fracture,
pneumonia

Normal
and/or
small effusion
and/or
small opacities

Treat appropriately

V/Q RADIONUCLIDE
SCAN

Normal

No embolism

V/Q Mismatch

Abnormal, but no
V/Q mismatch

High index
of suspicion

Low index
of suspicion

PULMONARY
ANGIOGRAM

Normal

Conservative
treatment

Abnormal

Pulmonary
embolism

Diagnostic decision tree 2

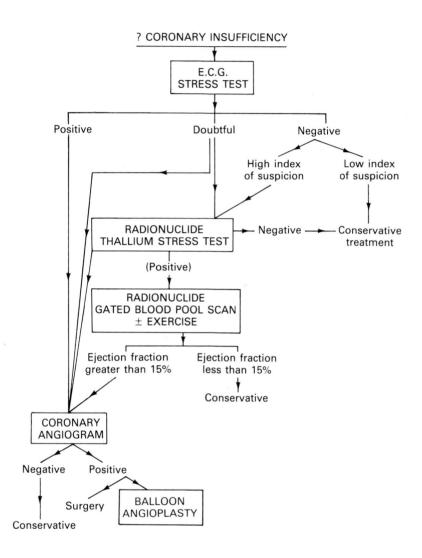

Diagnostic decision tree 3

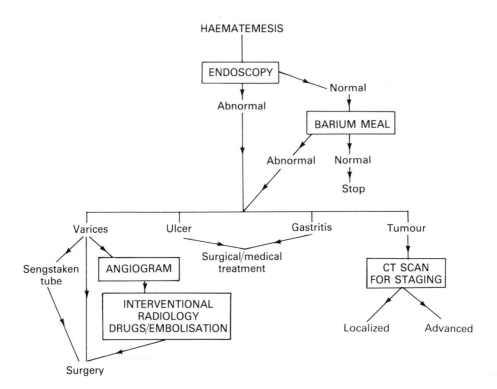

Diagnostic decision tree 4

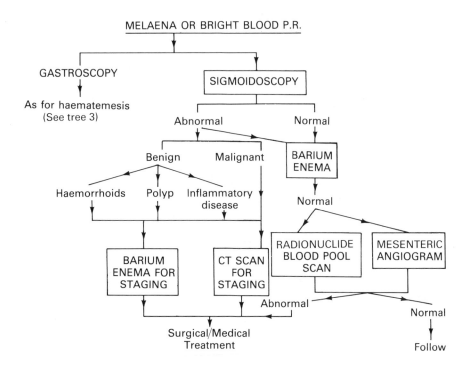

MELAENA OR BRIGHT BLOOD P.R.

GASTROSCOPY

As for haematemesis
(See tree 3)

SIGMOIDOSCOPY

Abnormal   Normal

Benign   Malignant

BARIUM ENEMA

Haemorrhoids   Polyp   Inflammatory disease

Normal

BARIUM ENEMA FOR STAGING

CT SCAN FOR STAGING

RADIONUCLIDE BLOOD POOL SCAN

MESENTERIC ANGIOGRAM

Abnormal

Surgical/Medical Treatment

Normal

Follow

Diagnostic decision tree 5

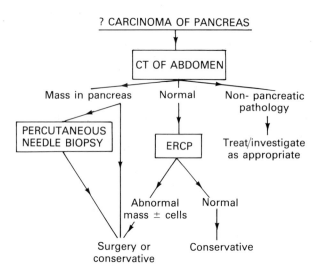

? CARCINOMA OF PANCREAS

CT OF ABDOMEN

Mass in pancreas — Normal — Non-pancreatic pathology

PERCUTANEOUS NEEDLE BIOPSY

ERCP

Treat/investigate as appropriate

Abnormal mass ± cells — Normal

Surgery or conservative

Conservative

Diagnostic decision tree 6a

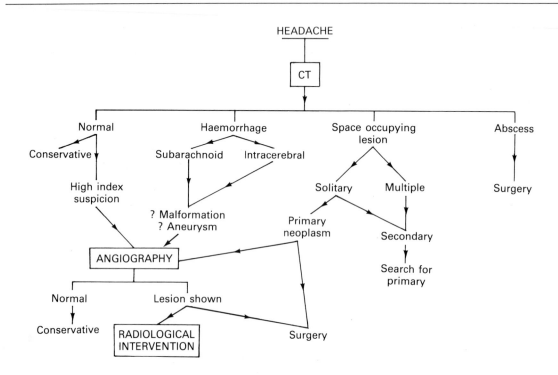

HEADACHE

CT

Normal — Haemorrhage — Space occupying lesion — Abscess

Conservative

Subarachnoid — Intracerebral

Solitary — Multiple

Surgery

High index suspicion

? Malformation ? Aneurysm

Primary neoplasm

Secondary

ANGIOGRAPHY

Search for primary

Normal — Lesion shown

Conservative

RADIOLOGICAL INTERVENTION

Surgery

Diagnostic decision tree 6b

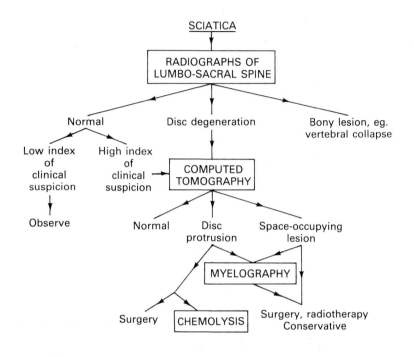

SCIATICA

RADIOGRAPHS OF
LUMBO-SACRAL SPINE

Normal   Disc degeneration   Bony lesion, eg.
                                       vertebral collapse

Low index   High index
of   of
clinical   clinical → COMPUTED
suspicion   suspicion   TOMOGRAPHY

Observe   Normal   Disc   Space-occupying
                     protrusion   lesion

MYELOGRAPHY

Surgery   CHEMOLYSIS   Surgery, radiotherapy
                                 Conservative

Diagnostic decision tree 6c

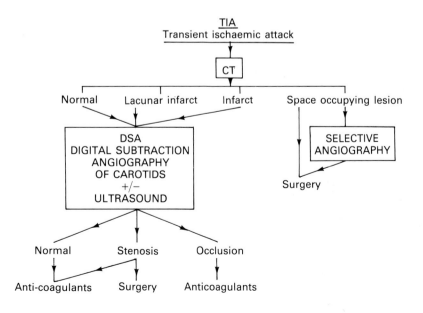

TIA
Transient ischaemic attack

CT

Normal   Lacunar infarct   Infarct   Space occupying lesion

DSA
DIGITAL SUBTRACTION
ANGIOGRAPHY
OF CAROTIDS
+/−
ULTRASOUND

SELECTIVE
ANGIOGRAPHY

Surgery

Normal   Stenosis   Occlusion

Anti-coagulants   Surgery   Anticoagulants

Diagnostic decision tree 7

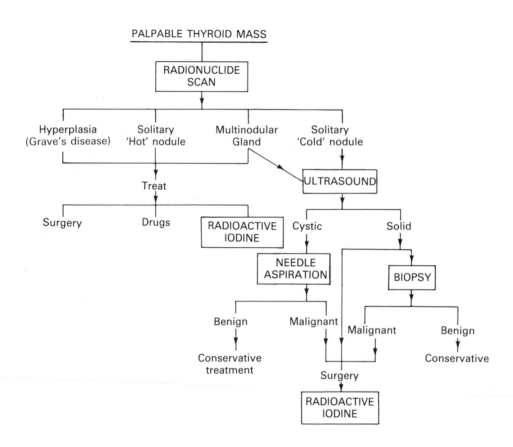

Diagnostic decision tree 8a

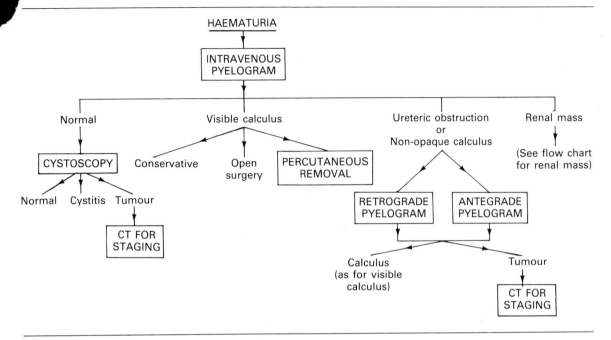

HAEMATURIA

INTRAVENOUS PYELOGRAM

Normal → CYSTOSCOPY → Normal / Cystitis / Tumour → CT FOR STAGING

Visible calculus → Conservative / Open surgery / PERCUTANEOUS REMOVAL

Ureteric obstruction or Non-opaque calculus → RETROGRADE PYELOGRAM / ANTEGRADE PYELOGRAM → Calculus (as for visible calculus) / Tumour → CT FOR STAGING

Renal mass → (See flow chart for renal mass)

Diagnostic decision tree 8b

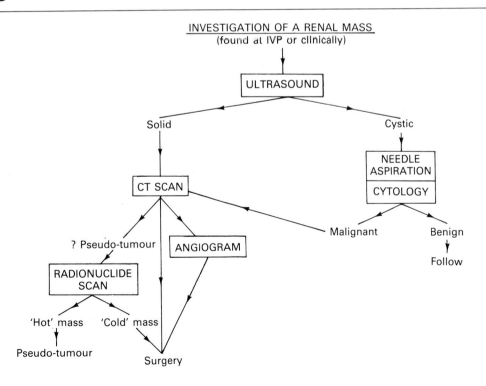

INVESTIGATION OF A RENAL MASS
(found at IVP or clinically)

ULTRASOUND

Solid → CT SCAN → ? Pseudo-tumour → RADIONUCLIDE SCAN → 'Hot' mass → Pseudo-tumour / 'Cold' mass → Surgery

ANGIOGRAM → Surgery

Cystic → NEEDLE ASPIRATION → CYTOLOGY → Malignant / Benign → Follow

Index